Peer Interventions for Health and Wellbeing

This book introduces peer interventions (primarily peer education, peer counselling and peer support) for the positive promotion of health and wellbeing as alternative or parallel methods to traditional clinical processes for reaching hard-to-access populations. It is strongly evidence-based, with chapters discussing reviews of the evidence, followed by important papers with key messages for implementation. Furthermore, it describes implementation and evaluation procedures, both in resource-rich environments and in developing countries.

Key Features:

- Bridges the traditional gap between professional clinical advice and the "real world", reaching where professionals cannot go
- Brings together information about those interventions that are well evidenced
- Distils information about how to implement interventions for medical professionals and paraprofessionals and charitable agencies and researchers
- Presents a fine balance between research and implementation, with evidence-driven guidance

Peer Interventions for Health and Wellbeing
Research into Practice

Keith James Topping

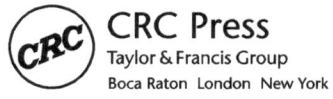

CRC Press
Taylor & Francis Group
Boca Raton London New York

CRC Press is an imprint of the
Taylor & Francis Group, an **informa** business

Designed cover image: Shutterstock.com

First edition published 2025
by CRC Press
2385 NW Executive Center Drive, Suite 320, Boca Raton FL 33431

and by CRC Press
4 Park Square, Milton Park, Abingdon, Oxon, OX14 4RN

CRC Press is an imprint of Taylor & Francis Group, LLC

This book contains information obtained from authentic and highly regarded sources. While all reasonable efforts have been made to publish reliable data and information, neither the author[s] nor the publisher can accept any legal responsibility or liability for any errors or omissions that may be made. The publishers wish to make clear that any views or opinions expressed in this book by individual editors, authors or contributors are personal to them and do not necessarily reflect the views/opinions of the publishers. The information or guidance contained in this book is intended for use by medical, scientific or health-care professionals and is provided strictly as a supplement to the medical or other professional's own judgement, their knowledge of the patient's medical history, relevant manufacturer's instructions and the appropriate best practice guidelines. Because of the rapid advances in medical science, any information or advice on dosages, procedures or diagnoses should be independently verified. The reader is strongly urged to consult the relevant national drug formulary and the drug companies' and device or material manufacturers' printed instructions, and their websites, before administering or utilizing any of the drugs, devices or materials mentioned in this book. This book does not indicate whether a particular treatment is appropriate or suitable for a particular individual. Ultimately it is the sole responsibility of the medical professional to make his or her own professional judgements, so as to advise and treat patients appropriately. The authors and publishers have also attempted to trace the copyright holders of all material reproduced in this publication and apologize to copyright holders if permission to publish in this form has not been obtained. If any copyright material has not been acknowledged, please write and let us know so we may rectify in any future reprint.

ISBN: 9781032572161 (hbk)
ISBN: 9781032572109 (pbk)
ISBN: 9781003438366 (ebk)

DOI: 10.1201/9781003438366

Typeset in Times LT Std
by KnowledgeWorks Global Ltd.
Access the Support Material: https://www.routledge.com/9781032572109

Contents

About the Author

Keith James Topping is Professor of Education at the University of Dundee Scotland and at RUDN University Moscow. He researches peer tutoring and peer assessment, computer-assisted learning and assessment, and artificial intelligence. He has over 470 publications in 19 languages, including multimedia in-service training and distance learning packs. He has degrees from the Universities of Sussex, Nottingham and Sheffield, and is a Fellow of the British Psychological Society. Former US President Bill Clinton cited him as an "outstanding researcher" for his input to the "America Reads" initiative. He was awarded the "Outstanding Contribution to Cooperative Learning Award" by the American Educational Research Association. He has consulted with national government and large organizations in several countries and researches and speaks all over the world (see https://en.wikipedia.org/wiki/Keith_James_Topping and https://discovery.dundee.ac.uk/en/persons/keith-topping).

Introduction

1

The aim of this book is to introduce peer intervention–peer education, peer counselling, and peer support–for the positive promotion of health and well-being as alternative or parallel methods to traditional professional clinical processes, especially for reaching hard-to-access populations. After defining the terms, book is intended to be strongly evidence-based, so each chapter proceeds to a discussion of reviews of the evidence on the effectiveness in that area, then often moves on to discuss key papers about particular projects that hold key messages for implementation. Each chapter then describes implementation procedures from one study in detail, to help practitioners who may well ask, "Yes, but how do we actually do it?"

Peer education, counselling, and support operate both in relatively resource-rich environments and also in developing countries. Consequently, the detailed description of the implementation of one program switches from a developed country to a less developed country by chapter, so readers can understand the problems of each. Even where resources are limited, implementation can often be improved by paying attention to simple organizational issues. The chapters are thus about half research evidence and half implementation details, but the implementation detail is directly drawn from the specific evidence given and directs readers to the original texts for more detail if they wish. The book is written in English with American spelling but is intended to have a global reach.

Arguably, peer education, peer counselling, and peer support have more chance of permeating the peer group and changing behavior than simple information-giving by professionals. A very important feature of these methods is that they can bridge the traditional gap between professional clinical advice and the "real world," reaching where professionals cannot be or cannot go. Many programs find gains for the helpers as well as the helped; to be a helper may actually be more therapeutic than being helped. Of course, peer education and counselling are not always a stand-alone program–quite often they are an integrated part of an initiative which also includes more traditional professional services.

DOI: 10.1201/9781003438366-1

Most of the literature on this subject is in peer-reviewed journal articles. This book brings together effectiveness information about those peer education, counselling, and support initiatives that are well evidenced and distils information about how to implement them. The evidence from diverse fields and the commonalities in implementation have never been brought together and explicated before.

This book is intended for relative newcomers to this field. Many medical personnel will have had training and experience that focuses on what they can do directly to help patients. This book takes a different angle—what can medical personnel do to train and support peers to work effectively with patients to support and guide them in a more informal way, often in a language they are more likely to understand, and often based on the helper's own experience of problems that is closely related to those the targeted person is suffering?

DEFINITIONS

Peer education can be defined as peers offering credible and reliable information about sensitive life issues which impact health and well-being and the opportunity to discuss them in a one-to-one or informal peer group setting.

Peer counselling can be defined as people from similar groupings who are not professionals who help to clarify life problems and identify solutions by listening; clarifying; feeding back; summarizing; questioning and being positive, supportive and reassuring and then helping plan, organize and problem-solve.

Peer support is more difficult to define, as it is widely used as an umbrella term with a degree of vagueness. Peer support occurs when people use their own experiences to help each other. It is intended to introduce the patient to ideas and approaches that others have found helpful and reassure the patient that they are not alone in how they are feeling. It aims to provide a space where patients feel accepted and understood and everyone's experiences are treated as being equally important, and involves both giving and receiving support. Peer support may involve meeting in person or can be accessed online—for example, through social media networks or communities, emails, phone calls, or text messages.

Occasionally, papers also refer to "peer mentoring," "peer navigation," and other terms. In all these cases, "peer" means someone of similar age and background who has no professional training in the area in question but may well have experienced the issues being discussed at firsthand. Peer educators, counsellors, and supporters of course should have benefited from some training to ensure the facts they are transmitting are accurate.

Peer education is usually done in groups, while peer counselling may be one-to-one, group-based, or a mixture of the two. Peer support is usually one-to-one. However, many authors make no attempt to define activities as one or the other, and indeed, peer education is sometimes very difficult to distinguish from peer counselling, while other authors refer simply to "peer support." As the terms peer education, counseling, and support are used very vaguely in the literature and are often interchangeable, no effort is made in the chapters to analyze them separately. We will return to this issue in chapter 15 and beyond. The intervening chapters focus on areas of application.

THEORY

Several theories have been invoked to explain the psychosocial benefits associated with peer support. These include: *social comparison theory*, which suggests people seek out the company of similar others to compare the appropriateness of their experiences and responses when under threat, resulting in normalizing effects, and *stress and coping theory*, which positions peer support as a coping resource which may buffer stress and suggests that the act of emotional expression can itself relieve stress. Additionally, the *helper therapy principle* notes that the helper's health and well-being benefit from helping another with a shared problem, suggesting that those who provide peer support may experience benefits, or from being able to assist others.

AUDIENCE

The primary audience for this book is medical professionals (doctors and nurses) and paraprofessionals, their associated senior undergraduate students and graduate students, and researchers and academics. The book could be supplementary/recommended reading for graduate courses. It is possible that managers of medical services seeking additional or alternative methods will also be interested in the book.

However, the book is not aimed at the inexperienced professional practitioner, who will be more concerned about honing their traditional skills.

Nor is it intended for practitioners in primary care, but rather for those working in secondary care. For example, engagement with general practitioners is not anticipated, as their brief is so wide and they are so busy. Also, the book is not aimed at peers actually delivering peer education and counselling on a day-to-day basis–their interests will be much more specific and concrete.

The primary audience for this book is thus pre- and in-service clinicians in public or private health and well-being services and their leaders and managers. In addition, clinicians working for charities or NGOs with a health and well-being orientation should be interested in the book. Those responsible for delivering training to such people will also be interested. This is likely to include many specialist doctors (who are likely to form the main readership for the book) but also senior nurses. The book is not only international but interdisciplinary and so might appeal to workers outside the medical profession also working to promote positive health and well-being, e.g., social workers, community workers, and psychologists. All of these should find the book valuable as a guide on implementing peer education and counselling projects successfully. Officials at local and national governments are also likely to use the book in determining policy, as will researchers. Perhaps even some politicians will be interested.

WHY READ THIS BOOK?

The book is intended to give the evidence base for peer intervention–peer education, peer counselling, and peer support programs and methods–in an easy, accessible, and comprehensible way. This should reassure readers that their practice or intended practice is well substantiated, so they can defend it when questioned. It also gives details of how methods can be implemented and refers readers to the original texts for more detail. Thus, readers are reassured that these methods work and are also given information about how to practically implement them.

SEARCH METHODS

Four relevant research databases (ERIC, Google Scholar, Medline, and Web of Science in that order) were searched for peer-reviewed journal papers using the terms: "peer education" OR "peer counselling" OR "peer counseling"

OR "peer support" AND (the title and/or subtitles of the chapter). Hits were extracted up to the point where ten consecutive pages in each database had no relevant hits. Campos et al. (2024) found that 95% of all relevant abstracts within a given dataset could be retrieved using heuristic stopping rules such as stopping the screening process after classifying 20% of records. Duplicates were excluded as the search moved from one database to the next. The fewest hits were found in ERIC, most hits were found in Google Scholar and Medline, and given this order, Web of Science struggled to generate new hits not otherwise found. Masters and doctoral theses were excluded, as their quality was so various. Books and chapters in books were also excluded on the grounds that they had also not been peer reviewed. Papers delivered at conferences were also excluded on grounds of uncertain quality.

The hits were read at the level of title and abstract. Papers were then selected which appeared to meet the inclusion criteria: written in the English language; peer-reviewed journal article; dated 2000 to present day; focusing on peer education, counselling, or support to promote health or well-being; being a systematic analysis or meta-analysis; or being a single study including quantitative and qualitative data to support the conclusions regarding effectiveness. After reading the full text of these papers, they were either selected or deselected. Each chapter indicates how many review and single-study papers were selected for that chapter (bearing in mind the order of database access and the rolling exclusions) although only a few single-study papers will be mentioned owing to constraints of space. In chapters where there are a great many review papers, the space given to single studies is necessarily smaller due to constraints of space. In chapters where there are few review papers, more space is given to single studies.

STRUCTURE OF THE BOOK

Many books which claim to be evidence-based just give vague background research which is often not reflected in the recommendations they make, but in the case of this book, the research cited is specifically about the method which is described. All of the chapters are supported by at least one review of research as well as many single studies. So far as the research is concerned, systematic reviews and meta-analyses will be reviewed first where they exist, followed by randomized controlled trials (RCTs) and other experimental and quasi-experimental research, and these are given the most detailed analysis.

The peer education, counselling, and support research falls into 13 categories, each with its own chapter: sexual health, HIV/AIDS, cancer (breast cancer and colorectal cancer screening), diabetes, other medical conditions (e.g., asthma, spinal cord injuries), mental health (general, depression, suicide prevention, schizophrenia), alcohol abuse, drug use, smoking, obesity and physical activity interventions, breastfeeding and nutrition, prisons, and other areas of interest.

The chapters follow a similar model: first, the area of interest is defined; then the relevant research is summarized by way of background, taking reviews first and then individual papers where space permits; then a specific program is chosen as an example, and its evidence summarized; and then its implementation is described in detail. A 13th chapter was added for a variety of other programs which were not evidenced by much literature but which might be of interest to those working in these less populated fields.

In some chapters, papers have been very approximately categorized into those reporting on developed countries and those reporting on developing countries since the contexts are often very different in different countries. However, this division is highly approximate, and the reader will sometimes find a paper reporting on a very disadvantaged group within a developed country categorized as a developing country (actually, a developing subgroup). Within the reporting here on single studies, attempts have been made to include studies from both developing and developed countries although the former are sometimes not as scientifically rigorous as the former. Additionally, regarding the specimen program selected for discussion, from one chapter to the next the focus alternates between papers from developing and developed countries.

These 13 chapters are prefaced by this Introduction which gives definitions and outlines common points of departure. They are followed by a further chapter which seeks to extract common implementation threads from the foregoing and emphasize features which are common to many programs. This should enable the reader to see the commonalities across the methods, which should help them devise their own methods and programs, and also highlight which of these features could be strengthened at little cost in developing countries. A yet further chapter addresses practical issues of evaluation, which are difficult but very necessary in this field. More than one method is of course desirable so that results can be triangulated. Finally, a discussion considers the relative strength of evidence in the preceding chapters and its implications for the future. Each chapter has its own references appended. As only a few single studies are discussed in each chapter, the references for all the other single studies that were found are in Appendix 1 (online only), but this is so long it is only available electronically on the book website: https://www.routledge.com/9781032572109.

The book is of slightly greater length than would be hoped for by most readers, but the sections most relevant to the reader can be read first (avoiding overstressing readers is desirable). The book thus offers a summary of the independent, peer-reviewed effectiveness research evidence on the methods described. This should address many of the major concerns of readers, who will have questions like "does it work?" "how should it be implemented to make it work?" and "is it cheaper and more efficient in time than what we were doing before?" This review of evidence should reassure readers that existing or intended practice is evidence-based and well substantiated, lead professionals to improve their implementation of such programs, and enable them to state and defend their case in that regard to managers, local and national governments, the general public, and other stakeholders. It will also be of interest to researchers, especially in areas where data are sparser or more difficult to track.

HOW TO READ THIS BOOK

Hopefully, the book is not too long for the busy person to find time to read at least some of it. Obviously, this Introductory chapter should be read first. After that, consider your context–are you working in a developing country or a more developed country? How restricted are you in terms of the time available and the willingness of your hierarchy to allow some innovation? If neither of these is positive, you might need to be subtle about how you introduce the peer activity. Then focus on which of chapters 2–14 is relevant to your special interest. Then you might read associated chapters which are somewhat relevant. The last chapters try to draw together the threads of commonality from all the previous sections and examine evaluation measures and may be useful for all to read after they have read the Introduction.

STATISTICAL ANALYSIS

Some (but not many) statistics are present in what follows, so here is a brief overview. The *number* of observations is usually indicated as n or N (this is important in terms of the size and consequently significance of the study). An arithmetic *mean* or *average is* the sum of all observations divided by the number of observations. The *standard deviation* (s.d.) is a measure of the amount of variance in the data. The correlation between two different variables is often expressed as a *correlation coefficient* (r), which indicates on a scale from −1 through 0 to + 1 whether the relationship is negative or positive and its degree.

In some analyses, you will see that the difference between sets of observations is tested for statistical significance. One way of doing this is with the *t-test*, which compares the means with reference to their s.d.s and ns and sees if the value of the resulting statistic t is large enough to be statistically significant. Other ways are more complicated to explain.

Statistical significance is a quantification of whether what you see is likely just due to random chance or whether it is more probably the result of some influential factor you are studying. Usually, a criterion of probability of 0.05 or 5% is set as the limit of statistical significance, below which what you see is more likely due to your factor of interest and above which it is more likely due to random chance. Sometimes the sample size (n) for an analysis is very large, and one result of this is that even very small differences appear statistically significant, as statistical significance is strongly affected by sample size–the larger the sample size, the more likely statistical significance becomes.

An alternative way of looking at this is via *effect size* (ES) (a quantitative measure of the magnitude of an effect). ESs are also known as *standardized mean difference* (SMD). The larger the ES, the stronger the relationship between two variables. ESs are often approximately categorized according to their size: very small = 0.01, small = 0.20, medium = 0.50, large = 0.80, very large = 1.20, huge = 2.00. There is another kind of ES (eta-squared: η^2) used occasionally, which we will talk about when it occurs.

OVERVIEWS OF EFFECTIVENESS– DOES IT WORK?

Although peer education, peer counselling, and peer support have been used very widely for over 50 years, for many of these years, the background research was weak. However, now the background research is strong in a number of areas, and these are the areas that this book concentrates on. There were many strong reviews, particularly in more recent years. Some were narrative, some were systematic analyses, and a few were meta-analyses. Some reviews focused on young people, others on adults, and some on a mixture of the two. Some were about preventive interventions, while others were about corrective interventions. Later reviews were more likely to include RCTs.

Some of these reviews found peer education or counselling to be as effective as or more effective than traditional professional clinical advice, at least in the populations under investigation. Some reviews were very broad and are summarized here rather than under later chapter headings. There were 26 such reviews in all. Fourteen of these were very broad in scope, and 12 were somewhat more focused, i.e., on adolescents (five reviews), schools (four), Indigenous youth (one), refugees (one), and vaccination (one).

Very Broad Reviews

Mellanby et al. (2000) evaluated school-based health education programs which compared the effects of peers or adults delivering the same material. Peer leaders were at least as effective as or more effective than adults. A systematic review was conducted by Harden et al. (2001), who found 210 studies with 64 (49 outcome evaluations and 15 process evaluations) meeting the inclusion criteria, predominantly from the USA. However, only 12 (24%) were judged methodologically sound. Four interventions focused on sexual health, five on the prevention of smoking, one on asthma education, one on violence prevention, and one on the prevention of testicular cancer. Of these, seven found the method to be effective for at least one behavioral outcome and three effective for nonbehavioral outcomes. Five studies compared the effectiveness of peers to other providers and found mixed results. Kim (2004) analyzed the efficacy of peer counseling in Korea from 1990 to 2003 using a meta-analysis of controlled studies, calculating 157 ESs from 36 studies. The average ES was 1.18. College students had the highest effects, followed by secondary students and elementary students.

The World Health Organization (2005) held a workshop on peer education in 2004, attended by WHO advisers from Bahrain, Egypt, Iraq, Jordan, Lebanon, Morocco, Oman, Saudi Arabia, Tunisia, and Yemen. The objectives of the workshop were to review success stories and elaborate guidelines to promote peer education, capacity building, follow-up, and evaluation. Webel et al. (2010) reviewed 25 randomized clinical trials. ESs ranged from −0.50 to 2.86. Peer-based interventions facilitated important changes in health-related behaviors, including physical activity, smoking, and condom use, with a small- to medium-sized effect. Interventions aimed at increasing breast-feeding, medication adherence, women's health screening, and participation in general activities did not produce significant changes. A meta-analysis was performed by Kang (2015) on 64 papers plus dissertations from 2000 to 2015, and 67 ESs were calculated. The average ES was 0.89.

Sokol and Fisher (2016) noted that hard-to-reach groups could be classified according to three domains: individual (e.g., psychological factors), demographic (e.g., socioeconomic status), and cultural–environmental (e.g., social network). They conducted three systematic searches in one database from 2000 to 2015. Forty-seven studies met the inclusion criteria and addressed eight health areas, including: maternal and child health (26%), diabetes (17%), and other chronic diseases (15%). Forty-four studies (94%) reported significant changes favoring peer support. Eleven strategies emerged for engaging and retaining participants. Programs that reported a strategy of trust and respect had a higher retention rate (83%) than programs not reporting such a strategy (48%; p = 0.003). Peer support benefits were greater among individuals characterized by disadvantage. A systematic review was conducted by Ramchand et al. (2017), who searched three databases for RCTs from 2005 to 2015 and found 116. In RCTs, there were more null than positive effects across peer interventions, with notable exceptions: group-based interventions that used peers as educators commonly improved knowledge, attitudes, beliefs, and perceptions and peer educators also commonly improved social health/connectedness and engagement. Dyadic peer support influenced behavior change, and peer counseling showed promising effects on physical health outcomes.

King and Simmons (2018) undertook a systematic review of randomized and non-randomized studies since 1995, including 37 studies. Outcomes that more often showed significant differences were patient activation, self-efficacy, empowerment, and hope. A scoping review was conducted by Lorthios-Guilledroit et al. (2018), who searched five databases and included 55 studies. Most studies ($n = 32$) used a qualitative research design. Health problems were mostly related to chronic diseases ($n = 19$) and HIV and sexually transmitted diseases ($n = 13$). Regarding implementation outcomes, most papers reported data on participants' responsiveness (i.e., participation rate, satisfaction, or engagement) ($n = 25$), peer leaders' responsiveness ($n = 23$), and program fidelity (mainly dose, i.e., proportion of the program that was delivered) ($n = 18$). However, the question of effectiveness was not really addressed. Haines et al. (2018) conducted a systematic search of four databases, screening 2932 studies but only including eight. The most common peer support model was an in-person, facilitated group for families that occurred during the patients' ICU admission. Peer support reduced psychological morbidity and improved social support and self-efficacy in two studies; in both, peer support was via an individual peer-to-peer model.

Madmoli et al. (2019) conducted a systematic review, searching six databases and including ten articles. Peer education led to increased self-care in diabetes and a reduction in anxiety in patients undergoing coronary artery bypass graft surgery. This type of training could be effective in many other diseases. Price et al. (2022) searched ten databases for systematic reviews, RCTs, and economic evaluations since 2015, including

91 studies: 32 systematic reviews, 52 RCTs, and seven economic evaluations. There were concentrations of evidence relating to different types of peer support, including education, psychological support, self-care/self-management, and social support. Most studies had been conducted in the USA. A rapid scoping review was conducted by Mikolajczak-Degrauwe et al. (2023), searching ten databases and including 45 studies, describing peer support initiatives among groups of young migrants and unsupervised minors, young adults with autism, people with mental health problems, foster/shelter families, vulnerable pregnant women, people outside the labor force, older adults, and homeless people. The strength of peer support was its positive effect on the quality of life among vulnerable people. Opportunities included mutual learning, anticipated long-term effects, and facilitation of social inclusion.

More Focused Reviews

Five papers concerned adolescents. Abdi and Simbar (2013) searched three databases from 1999 to 2013. Peer education seemed effective in promoting healthy behaviors among adolescents although not all programs were successful. A narrative review was offered by Azizi et al. (2017), who searched six databases from 1991 to 2016 and included 53 articles but described characteristics of programs rather than outcomes. Araujo (2018) reported on Youth Health Champions across Europe, a role which harnessed young people's inclination to seek and use peer support to address issues, concerns, and general decisions. A literature review included training manuals published by a number of organizations including the United Nations Population Fund (UNFPA), the Guide Association, Lund University in Sweden, the European Commission and also 15 case studies of projects from across Europe. Peer education was a widely used approach. There was strong evidence that peer education increased healthier lifestyles. Iranian adolescents were the focus of Ghasemi et al. (2019), who searched eight databases from 2000 to 2018 and included 20 articles on the effects in the prevention of disease, mental health, nutritional behaviors, and prevention of high-risk behaviors. In all categories, the results showed an equal or greater effect of peer education on knowledge, attitude, practice, self-efficacy, and health behavior of adolescents compared to other methods such as education by teacher, health personnel, lecture, pamphlet, and booklet. Rose-Clarke et al. (2019) specifically focused on adolescents in low- and middle-income countries, searching for RCTs across infectious and vaccine preventable diseases, undernutrition, HIV/AIDS, sexual and reproductive health, unintentional injuries, violence, physical disorders, mental disorders, and substance use in a narrative review of 20 studies.

Fourteen studies were linked to schools or colleges. Eleven studies reported positive outcomes. Four studies reported initiatives in a school base, which would have different organizational features from a community-based project and might include primary as well as secondary pupils.

Petosa and Smith (2014) conducted a systematic review and found "peer mentoring" effective for promoting health behavior change. It allowed for the incorporation of skill-building activities, reinforcement of self-regulation activities, engagement in individual and group activities, and receiving social support to meet personal health goals. Twelve databases were searched by Shackleton et al. (2016) after 1980, who included 22 reviews. Multicomponent interventions (including school policy changes, parent involvement, and work with local communities) were effective for promoting sexual health and preventing bullying and smoking. There was less evidence that such intervention could reduce alcohol and drug use. King and Fazel (2021) searched 11 databases for a systematic review, including 11 studies, showing that peer-led interventions had been used to address a range of mental health and well-being issues. Two studies out of seven that investigated peer leaders showed significant improvements in self-esteem and social stress. Two studies out of five that investigated recipient outcomes showed significant improvements in self-confidence and quality of life measure, with one study showing a decrease in mental health scores. Five databases were searched by Dodd et al. (2022) to 2020, and 73 articles were included. The majority of papers focused on sex education/HIV prevention ($n = 23$), promoting healthy lifestyles ($n = 17$), and alcohol, smoking, and substance use ($n = 16$). Of 67 papers reporting recipient outcomes, 52% showed evidence of effectiveness, 12% (8 out of 67) showed mixed findings, and 36% found limited or no evidence of effectiveness. Improvement in health-related knowledge was most common with less evidence for positive health behavior change.

One paper on Indigenous youth was offered by Vujcich et al. (2018), who searched three databases and included 24 studies (all Australian or North American). Only one was an RCT. Outcomes included improved knowledge, attitude, and behaviors. The literature was dominated by Australian sexual health interventions. Salem-Pickartz (2007) focused on refugees, having trained 49 peer counsellors in two refugee camps, and gave an overview of the training content and strategies. The main components of a culturally sensitive, client-centered empowerment approach to psychosocial intervention in a situation of continuous deprivation and insecurity were outlined. Gobbo et al. (2023) focused on vaccination, conducting a systematic search of two databases up to 2022 and including 16 articles. Half of the studies had students as their population. The human papillomavirus vaccine was the most common vaccine assessed, followed by COVID-19 and influenza vaccines. Eleven out of 16 articles reported a positive impact, and two studies had mixed results.

WHAT THE BOOK IS NOT

The approaches mentioned in the chapters that follow have been found to be effective, and the research on them is briefly summarized. However, there are many other programs and methods which have not been widely evaluated or not evaluated at all. We do not mention these approaches further in this book.

REFERENCES

Abdi, F., & Simbar, M. (2013). The peer education approach in adolescents - narrative review article. *Iranian Journal of Public Health*, *42*(11), 1200–1206.

Araujo, N. (2018). Reviewing the evidence of effective peer education among young people. *Perspectives in Public Health*, *138*(6), 299–300. https://doi.org/10.1177/1757913918801472

Azizi, M., Hamzehgardeshi, Z., & Shahhosseini, Z. (2017). Influential factors for the improvement of peer education in adolescents: A narrative review. *Journal of Pediatrics Review*, *5*(1), 38–44. http://jpr.mazums.ac.ir/article-1-135-en.html

Campos, D. G. et al. (2024). Screening smarter, not harder: A comparative analysis of machine learning screening algorithms and heuristic stopping criteria for systematic reviews in educational research. *Educational Psychology Review*, *36*(19). https://doi.org/10.1007/s10648-024-09862-5

Dodd, S., Widnall, E., Russell, A. E., Curtin, E. L., Simmonds, R., Limmer, M., & Kidger, J. (2022). School-based peer education interventions to improve health: A global systematic review of effectiveness. *BMC Public Health*, *22*, 2247. https://doi.org/10.1186/s12889-022-14688-3

Ghasemi, V., Simbar, M., Rashidi Fakari, F., Saei Ghare Naz, M., & Kiani, Z. (2019). The effect of peer education on health promotion of Iranian adolescents: A systematic review. *International Journal of Pediatrics*, *7*(3), 9139–9157. https://doi.org/10.22038/ijp.2018.36143.3153

Gobbo, E. L. S., Hanson, C., Abunnaja, K. S. S., & van Wees, S. H. (2023). Do peer-based education interventions effectively improve vaccination acceptance? A systematic review. *BMC Public Health*, *23*, 1354. https://doi.org/10.1186/s12889-023-16294-3

Haines, K. J., Beesley, S. J., Hopkins, R. O., McPeake, J., Quasim, T., Ritchie, K., & Iwashyna, T. J. (2018). Peer support in critical care: A systematic review. *Critical Care Medicine*, *46*(9), 1522–1531. https://doi.org/10.1097/CCM.0000000000003293

Harden, A., Oakley, A., & Olive, S. (2001). Peer-delivered health promotion for young people: A systematic review of different study designs. *Health Education Journal, 60*(4), 339–353. https://doi.org/10.1177/001789690106000406

Kang, G. M. (2015). Meta-analysis of effect of peer counseling program on adolescents. *Journal of Future Oriented Youth Society, 12*(3), 87–110.

Kim, K. H. (2004). A meta-analysis on the effectiveness of peer counseling conducted in Korea. *The Korea Journal of Youth Counseling, 12*(2), 3–10.

King, T., & Fazel, M. (2021). Examining the mental health outcomes of school-based peer-led interventions on young people: A scoping review of range and a systematic review of effectiveness. *PLoS ONE, 16*(4), e0249553. https://doi.org/10.1371/journal.pone.0249553

King, A. J., & Simmons, M. B. (2018). A systematic review of the attributes and outcomes of peer work and guidelines for reporting studies of peer interventions. *Psychiatric Services, 69*, 961–977. https://doi.org/10.1176/appi.ps.201700564

Lorthios-Guilledroit, A., Lucie, R., & Filiatrault, J. (2018). Factors associated with the implementation of community-based peer-led health promotion programs: A scoping review. *Evaluation and Program Planning, 68*, 19–33. https://doi.org/10.1016/j.evalprogplan.2018.01.008

Madmoli, M., Khodadadi, M., Papi Ahmadi, F., & Niksefat, M. (2019). A systematic review on the impact of peer education on self-care behaviors of patients. *International Journal of Health and Biological Sciences, 2*(1), 1–5. https://doi.org/10.30750/ IJHBS.2.1.1

Mellanby, A. R., Rees, J. B., & Tripp, J. H. (2000). Peer-led and adult-led school health education: A critical review of available comparative research. *Health Education Research, 15*(5), 533–545. https://doi.org/10.1093/her/15.5.533

Mikolajczak-Degrauwe, K. et al. (2023). Strengths, weaknesses, opportunities and threats of peer support among disadvantaged groups: A rapid scoping review. *International Journal of Nursing Sciences, 10*(4), 587–601. https://doi.org/10.1016/j.ijnss.2023.09.002

Petosa, R. L., & Smith, L. H. (2014). Peer mentoring for health behavior change: A systematic review. *American Journal of Health Education, 45*(6), 351–357. https://doi.org/10.1080/19325037.2014.945670

Price, A., de Bell, S., Shaw, N., Bethel, A., Anderson, R., & Coon, J. T. (2022). What is the volume, diversity and nature of recent, robust evidence for the use of peer support in health and social care? An evidence and gap map. *Campbell Systematic Reviews, 18*(3), e1264. https://doi.org/10.1002/cl2.1264

Ramchand, R., Ahluwalia, S. C., Xenakis, L., Apaydin, E., Raaen, L., & Grimm, G. (2017). A systematic review of peer-supported interventions for health promotion and disease prevention. *Preventive Medicine, 101*, 156–170. https://doi.org/10.1016/j.ypmed.2017.06.008

Rose-Clarke, K., Bentley, A., Marston, C., & Prost, A. (2019). Peer-facilitated community-based interventions for adolescent health in low- and middle-income countries: A systematic review. *PLoS ONE, 14*(1): e0210468. https://doi.org/10.1371/journal.pone.0210468

Salem-Pickartz, J. (2007). Peer counsellors training with refugees from Iraq: A Jordanian case study. *Intervention, 5*(3), 232–243.

Shackleton, N., Jamal, F., Viner, R., Dickson, K., Patton, G., & Bonell, C. (2016). School-based interventions going beyond health education to promote adolescent health:

Systematic review of reviews. *Journal of Adolescent Health, 58*(4), 382–396. https://www.sciencedirect.com/science/article/pii/S1054139X15007363

Sokol, R., & Fisher, E. (2016). Peer support for the hardly reached: A systematic review. *American Journal of Public Heath, 106*, e1–e8. https://doi.org/10.2105/AJPH.2016.303180

Vujcich, D., Thomas, J., Crawford, K., & Ward, J. (2018). Indigenous youth peer-led health promotion in Canada, New Zealand, Australia, and the United States: A systematic review of the approaches, study designs, and effectiveness. *Frontiers in Public Health, 6*, e1–e8. https://doi.org/10.3389/fpubh.2018.00031

Webel, A. R., Okonsky, J., Trompeta, J., & Holzemer, W. L. (2010). A systematic review of the effectiveness of peer-based interventions on health-related behaviors in adults. *American Journal of Public Health, 100*, 247–253. https://doi.org/10.2105/AJPH.2008.149419

World Health Organization (2005). *Adolescent peer education in formal and non-formal settings. Report of an inter-country workshop.* Cairo: WHO.

Sexual Health

2

DEFINITION

Sexual health is defined as:

- Enjoyment of sexual relations without exploitation, oppression, or abuse.
- Safe pregnancy and childbirth, and avoidance of unintended pregnancies.
- Absence and avoidance of sexually transmitted infections, including HIV.

Sexual health is a state of physical, emotional, mental, and social well-being in relation to sexuality. It is not merely the absence of disease, dysfunction, or infirmity. Sexual health includes a sense of self-esteem, personal attractiveness, and competence, as well as freedom from sexual dysfunction, sexually transmitted diseases, and sexual assault/coercion. Sexual health at the least involves freedom from unwanted sexual intercourse, freedom from sexually transmitted infections (STIs), and freedom from unwanted pregnancy. STIs such as bacterial vaginosis, chlamydia, trichomonas, hepatitis, genital herpes, gonorrhea, and syphilis can be problems. The most significant risk factor for cervical cancer is the human papillomavirus (an STI). Either gender can suffer from too little or too much libido. For men, premature ejaculation or erectile dysfunction can be problems. In developing countries, avoiding unwanted pregnancy (especially in young girls) and STIs are key issues.

There is a clear relationship between sexual ill health, poverty, and social exclusion. There is also an unequal impact of STI infection on gay men and certain minority ethnic groups. There have been large increases in many STIs in the last 10 years, including chlamydia (up 300%), gonorrhea (up 200%), and HIV (up 300%). Since 1990, people are having sex for the first time at a younger age; a greater proportion of people have multiple partners; and a

16   DOI: 10.1201/9781003438366-2

greater proportion of men report having had a same-sex partner. As many symptoms are asymptomatic, and many cases don't present due to stigma, the infection statistics are likely to be just the tip of the iceberg. Co-infections are often common, and an infection with an STI makes transmission of HIV easier.

REVIEWS OF EVIDENCE

There were 19 reviews of evidence. Six of these were concerned with youth and adolescence, five with school- and college-based programs, four with developing countries (general, Iran, India, and Southeast Asia), three with LGBT populations, and one with digital sexual health.

Sexual Health for Youth and Adolescence

United Nations Educational, Scientific and Cultural Organization (2003) offered an early review of the wealth of educational resources that already existed in adolescent sexual health. Their report also focused on what the research said was the impact of peer education in promoting changes in attitudes and behavior. This report synthesizes practical experiences and shares lessons learned. A systematic review by Kim and Free (2008) searched for quasi-randomized and randomized controlled trials of peer-led adolescent sexual health education 1998–2005. Thirteen articles met the inclusion criteria. No effects on condom use were found. One study reported a reduced risk of chlamydia (effect size 0.2), but another found no impact on STI incidence. One study found that young women (but not young men) were more likely to not have had sex. However, most interventions produced improvements in knowledge, attitudes, and intentions.

Tolli (2012) focused on pregnancy and HIV prevention in European studies, systematically reviewing from 1999 to 2010. Only five studies were selected. A few statistically significant changes were observed, but overall, there was no clear evidence of effectiveness concerning HIV prevention, adolescent pregnancy prevention, and sexual health promotion. Evaluating peer-led sexual health education interventions in more developed countries was the aim of Sun et al. (2018). Five databases were searched and 15 articles were selected. The majority of articles found improvements in sexual health knowledge (13 of 14) and attitudes (11 of 15). Two studies showed improved self-efficacy, and three showed behavioral changes. Meta-analysis revealed a large effect on knowledge change (effect size = 0.84) and a medium effect on attitude change (0.49).

Mahat and Scoloveno (2018) focused on HIV/STI risk, searching five databases from 2000 to 2016. Thirty articles were included. There was evidence of the effectiveness of programs on knowledge, attitudes, normative beliefs, and self-efficacy. However, the studies were equivocal on changes in sexual behavior. Peer educators and learners placed a high value on peer-led programs. Low and middle-income countries were the focus of Fantaye et al. (2022), who searched 11 databases from 2000 to 2020 and extracted 11 eligible articles. There was evidence of significant intervention effects on protective knowledge, attitudes, behaviors, and skills for preventing sexual violence and HIV infection. The strongest evidence was for improvement in knowledge.

Sexual Health on School and College Campuses

A review from Indonesia by Pusmaika and Novianti (2017) focused on school-based programs. They searched five databases and included seven studies. The majority showed that such programs had shown positive impact. Wong et al. (2019) reviewed programs on college campuses, including eight articles. Peer education was beneficial for increasing knowledge of sexual health topics and creating some behavior changes, such as increased condom use and HIV testing. Additionally, interventions developed specifically for women were effective. Five databases were searched by Dodd et al. (2022) to 2020, who included 73 studies. Papers mainly reported peer learner outcomes, with only six papers focusing solely on peer educator outcomes and five papers examining both peer learner and peer educator outcomes. Of the 67 papers reporting peer learner outcomes, 35/67 (52.2%) showed evidence of effectiveness, 8/67 (11.9%) showed mixed findings, and 24/67 (35.8%) found limited or no evidence of effectiveness. Improvement in health-related knowledge was most common, with less evidence for positive health behavior change.

Niland and Nearchou (2023) systematically reviewed the evidence on effectiveness, particularly behavior change techniques. Twenty-seven studies met the inclusion criteria. Studies examined sexual health behaviors such as condom usage, frequency of sexual activity, initiation of sexual activity, and number of sexual partners. Nine behavior change techniques were identified, with the most used being information about health consequences and social and emotional consequences, demonstration of behavior, behavioral practice/rehearsal, and instructions on how to perform the behavior. School-based sex education interventions could be effective in promoting positive sexual health behaviors. College campus sexual assault prevention programs were studied by Kettrey et al. (2023), who noted they were required by federal law. They conducted a systematic review including 385 effect sizes from 80 eligible studies from 1991 to 2021. Such programs had more effect on attitudes/knowledge than actual violence. Effects on sexual assault victimization were significant but small (effect size 0.15). The use of a risk reduction framework seemed to reduce effectiveness.

Sexual Health in Developing Countries

An early review by Price and Knibbs (2009) offered a critique of peer education programs in developing countries. Peer education was more complex and problematic than its popularity implied. The often-simplistic model of social relations that underlay peer education interventions led to the reinforcement of gendered power relations and a failure to take account of the social dynamics of poverty. However, the appeal of the approach remained powerful, stemming from engaging young people in health interventions in a way that increased their autonomy and capacity. This article reviewed very little evidence.

Farahani (2020) reviewed the evidence on the sexual and reproductive health of young people in Iran from 2001 to 2019. Forty-three articles were included. Although the majority of youth abstained from sex before marriage, significant minorities were sexually active before marriage, with a huge heterogeneity based on gender and geographical region. Multiple partners, inconsistent condom use, and younger age at sexual debut were more prevalent among men than women. Peer education programs in India were studied by Siddiqui et al. (2020). A systematic review included 13 articles. Peer education was implemented as part of multi-component programs and as a stand-alone intervention. The outcomes were mixed; some initiatives found significant outcomes and others did not.

Newman et al. (2022) investigated programs in Southeast Asia, conducting a scoping review to identify key characteristics, implementation challenges and knowledge, and identifying 17 peer-reviewed articles from Thailand ($n = 7$), Vietnam ($n = 5$), Myanmar ($n = 3$), Cambodia ($n = 1$), and Laos ($n = 1$). Benefits and challenges were evident. Knowledge gaps emerged in regard to peer educator outcomes (increased knowledge, skill-building, empowerment); interpersonal processes between peer educators and young people (role modeling, social dynamics); and social-structural contexts (sociocultural influences, gendered power relations).

Sexual Health for LGBT Populations

Ye et al. (2014) reviewed the effectiveness of peer interventions to reduce unprotected anal intercourse among men who have sex with men. Thirteen databases were searched up to 2012, and 22 studies were included. Peer-led interventions reduced unprotected anal intercourse with any sexual partners (mean effect size = 0.27). Heterogeneity was large.

The perspectives of both youth and facilitators on the delivery and receipt of LGBTI + (Lesbian, Gay, Bisexual, Transgender, Intersex) inclusive sexual health education were investigated by O'Farrell et al. (2021). A systematic review searched three online databases from 1990 to 2021, including 24 studies. The majority noted that both LGBTI+ youth and those who facilitate sexual health education were turning to online sources of information. Current programs operated from a heterosexual perspective, creating a sense of exclusion for LGBTI + youth. This was compounded by a lack of training, resulting in facilitators feeling ill-equipped or inhibited by their personal biases.

Freestone et al. (2022) studied both gay and bisexual men who had sex with men, searching five databases and including 38 studies. There were four intervention modalities: peer counselling [n = 6], groupwork programs [n = 15], peer navigation [n = 7], and peer education [n = 10]. Most addressed HIV, and evaluations demonstrated compelling evidence of significant effect across intervention modalities.

Digital Sexual Health

Martin et al. (2020) studied sexual health promotion for adolescents and young adults on the Internet. Web-based participatory interventions were thought to have potential in view of the internet's popularity among young people. A systematic review searched two databases and selected 60 articles, which described 37 interventions. Effectiveness results were less common than process results. Many of the 37 interventions were developed on websites (n = 20). The second most used medium was online social networks (n = 13), with Facebook dominating this group (n = 8). Another participatory component was game-type activity (n = 10). Videos were used by more than half of the interventions (n = 20). Less than half of the interventions had been evaluated (n = 17), while one-third (n = 12) reported plans to do so. Sexual behaviors were the most evaluated (n = 14), followed by condom use (n = 11), and sexual health knowledge (n = 8).

SINGLE STUDIES

Number of Single Studies

There were 87 single studies, 39 in developed countries and 48 (55%) in developing countries, reflecting the degree of concern in developing countries. As the reviews were so numerous, there was only space for two single studies.

Exemplar Single Studies Developed Context

Wilson et al. (2016) conducted a randomized controlled trial (RCT) on peer counselling with respect to contraception. The aim was to evaluate the impact peer counselling had on desire for long-acting, reversible contraception (LARC) among adolescents attending a family planning clinic. A randomized, controlled trial of 110 adolescent females attending an outpatient clinic for contraception were the participants, who received either brief peer counselling about LARC with routine contraceptive counselling, or routine counselling alone. Peer counselling was well received, and 70% of participants reported that it was helpful in contraceptive decision-making. Peer counselling did not affect same-day desire for LARC, but those who received the intervention were more likely to report increased knowledge and positive change in attitudes toward LARC. Positive factors included greater reported peer contraceptive influence, peer use of LARC, and social support. Twenty of the 36 adolescents desired LARC at the end of their clinic visit.

Exemplar Single Studies Developing Context

Peer education is an intervention within the voluntary medical male circumcision (VMMC) and Adolescent Sexual Reproductive Health linkages projects in Bulawayo and Mount Darwin, Zimbabwe (Mangombe et al., 2020). Little was known about whether results extended beyond increasing knowledge. The authors, therefore, assessed the extent of and factors affecting referral by peer educators and receipt of HIV testing services (HTS), contraception, management of STIs, and VMMC services by young people (10–24 years) counselled. This was a cohort study involving all young people counselled by 95 peer educators during three months, through secondary analysis of routinely collected data. Factors (clients' age, gender, marital and schooling status, counselling type, location, and peer educators' age and gender) affecting non-referral and non-receipt of services (dependent variables) were assessed. Of the 3370 counselled (66% men), 65% were referred for at least one service, and 58% of men were referred for VMMC. Other services had 5%–13% referrals. Counselling by men and rural locations reduced the risk of non-referral for VMMC, while age increased it. Receipt of services was high (64%–80%) except for STI referrals (39%). Rural location increased the risk of non-receipt of contraception, while marriage reduced it.

SPECIFIC PROGRAM

Mitchell et al. (2020) described a program in secondary schools in the UK. Young people report higher levels of unsafe sex and have higher rates of sexually transmitted infections than any other age group. Schools are well placed to facilitate early intervention. The authors report the Sexually Transmitted infections And Sexual Health (STASH) intervention in six schools with students aged 14–16 years. Control data were provided by students in the year above the intervention group. STASH involved peer nomination to identify the most influential students as peer supporters, aiming to recruit and train 15% of the year group. They delivered sexual health messages to friends in their year group via conversations and the use of Facebook to share varied content from a curated set of web-based resources. Peer supporters were themselves given support via follow-up sessions and trainer membership in Facebook groups.

Effectiveness

Data sources included a peer supporter questionnaire; observations of activities; interviews with trainers, teachers, peer supporters, and students; a monitoring log of peer supporter activities (including on Facebook and meeting attendance); a questionnaire to the control year group (covering baseline characteristics, social networks, mediators, and sexual health outcomes); a baseline and a follow-up questionnaire (approximately six months later) for the intervention year group. A total of 104 students were trained as peer supporters (just over half of those nominated for the role by their peers). Role retention was very high (97%). Of 611 students completing the follow-up questionnaire, 58% reported exposure to STASH activities. Intervention acceptability was high among students and stakeholders. Activities were delivered with good fidelity. The peer supporters were active, representative of their year group, and well-connected within their social network. A primary outcome of 'always safer sex' was identified, measured as no sex or always condom use for vaginal or anal sex in the last six months. The intervention cost £42 per student. The STASH intervention was feasible and acceptable in a UK secondary school.

Implementation

The aim was to reduce transmission of STIs and improve the sexual health of secondary school students aged 14–16 years. Professional trainers were used to train peer supporters to increase intervention efficacy and credibility, and reduce the burden on schools.

The authors sought to identify the most influential students in the target year by blind peer nomination. From this influential group, they intended to recruit a percentage of the entire year group to act as PSs.

Motivating Schools

School buy-in would be key to successful implementation. Helping schools meet national policy requirements would be a strong motivator. This related particularly to the Scottish Government's Curriculum for Excellence, Getting It Right for Every Child policy, and the National Health and Wellbeing Outcomes. The brochure for schools therefore explicitly outlined how the intervention could help schools meet relevant indicators, particularly around enhancing students' confidence and sense of responsibility, and addressing stigmatizing attitudes.

Pilot Consultations

Initial consultations with young people involved 16 participants aged 14–19 years. Three group interviews (20 participants in total) were conducted with young people outside the intervention area. Two group interviews were school-based, and the third was with a community center-based youth group (conducted at a community center).

Feedback

The literature suggested that young people's sexual health knowledge tends to converge around risk, STIs, and contraception, and that current gaps included communication, consent, pornography, sexual pleasure, and online literacy. Stakeholder consultation highlighted that current packages were outdated and lacked information on contemporary issues, such as consent and coercion, a view echoed in the young people consultations. Young people also expressed a desire for relatable experiential information and, echoing the literature, suggested that the use of humor and interactive components would enhance training and online content.

Resources

The authors collated high-quality resource exemplars (websites, resource packs). They sought to identify key features and identify potentially relevant content. Resources were categorized by source, type and quality, and key points were summarized. The quality of youth-oriented sexual health web resources was assessed (including information sites, YouTube videos, and vloggers/influencers), rating them according to relevance, content quality, design quality (appeal to young people), and apparent authority or legitimacy.

Media Platforms

Candidate social media platforms were reviewed for user demographics, functionality, appeal, and regulatory information. Platforms (e.g., Instagram, WhatsApp, Snapchat, and Facebook) were appraised for age restrictions, message-sharing functions (including traceability over time, images, audio, video, and ability to interface with a website), private group messaging options, and whether or not posted content could be visible to the research team to enable evaluation. The review of platforms suggested the following priorities for functionality: appeal to young people; provide options to post web links, images, and/or text; provide an option to create private, invite-only groups; ease of viewing messages and message stability; potential for monitoring; and potential for interface with a website. This ruled out popular platforms such as Snapchat (messages disappear, primarily images) and Twitter (messages likely to be lost in traffic, primarily appeals to older users). Instagram (primarily visual) at the time had no option for private groups or for a bespoke application programming interface to link to the study website. WhatsApp was ruled out on the basis that this would necessitate participants sharing mobile telephone numbers with fellow group members. We also ruled out school-linked platforms, such as Glow (https://glowconnect.org.uk/), which might limit credibility and perceived student ownership of the project. Ultimately, Facebook was identified as the only platform to meet all priorities.

Website

An interactive website and content management system was developed to provide mobile-optimized access, desktop functionality, and multilevel access for use by supporters and trainers, and the research team. Two school-based groups were visited to gauge opinions on draft website content. Participants reviewed drafts (via tablet and smartboard) and gave views on visual appeal and ease of use, topics and messages, language, acceptability of external links, information gaps, and general acceptability. Five students took part in brief cognitive interviews to test selected questionnaire items. Workshops were conducted in school time, lasted approximately 1.5 hours, and were audio-recorded. The research team then worked to streamline and simplify content and structure, and improve visual appeal, primarily via the creation of bespoke infographics. Group interviews were conducted with two youth groups: one face-to-face with an established young people's action research group and one online using Facebook Messenger. Groups comprising six (all female) and seven (four female, three male) participants, respectively. Groups discussed relevance, credibility, and relatability of newly created content.

Among the resources were two key videos that conveyed experiential information and behavior modeling. 'Ryan and Natalie' used a gently comedic approach to illustrate a young couple navigating their first sexual encounter (www.truetube.co.uk/film/Screwball), while 'Tea and Consent' (https://www.youtube.com/watch?v=pZwvrxVavnQ) also used humor and a tea metaphor to explain sexual consent. Hannah Witton was identified as an important 'influencer' (https://hannahwitton.com), and the BISH (Best in Sexual Health) website had a strong appeal to young people (www.bishuk.com). The final version of the website only required a school-wide password (circulated by supporters). Opening the website to all students could allow supporters to direct friends to visit for themselves. Key revisions of the website included the removal of subsections for different activity types, replacing textual messages with more visually appealing bespoke infographics and memes, reducing external links (participants tended not to click on these), and dropping conversation prompts (which were minimally engaged with). 'Gamifying' the online component was proposed as a means of boosting interactivity, engagement, and motivation, but was ultimately dropped in favor of simplicity.

Participants in website testing groups were positive about the revised website, particularly with the inclusion of humorous memes and brightly colored visuals. The final version of the STASH study website (www.stashtrial.org.uk) was organized under eight topics:

1. What's STASH all about?
2. Is my relationship good?
3. What's normal?
4. Am I ready for sex?
5. What's consent?
6. How do I avoid risk?
7. Are pics and porn OK?
8. How do I feel good about myself?

Each topic had a website page, comprising an overview and a series of easily sharable messages (text, memes, infographics, embedded videos, external links).

Peer Nomination

Peer nomination (as opposed to teacher or self-selection) would identify the most 'credible' or 'trustworthy' students and schools should not be allowed to shape the list of peer-nominated students. This was stipulated in the guidance provided to schools. All students in the target year (aged 14–16 years) were asked to complete a peer nomination questionnaire. Nomination questions included:

1. Who do you respect in your year at your school?
2. Who are good leaders in sports or other group activities in your year?
3. Who do you look up to in your year?'
4. With whom in your year would you feel comfortable talking about something personal or sensitive?
5. Who in your year is good at encouraging and persuading others to do things?
6. Whose opinion do you trust and value most in your year?
7. Who in your year is confident at talking to people outside their friendship group?

The 25% of young people receiving most nominations, stratified by gender, were invited to a recruitment meeting.

Training

A two-day supporter training session was held in school time, at an external venue, facilitated by external agencies. It was intended to equip peer supporters (PSs) with the knowledge, skills, and confidence required for the role; build motivation and enthusiasm for the role; generate trust and rapport within the group; build sexual health knowledge and skills; improve understanding of risks and consequences; build self-esteem and self-efficacy; reinforce social support for healthy sexual norms; and boost intrinsic motivation and autonomy. Supporters were required to sign a code of conduct during training and agree on a plan to 'announce' the project to their year group. Trainer-led activities also included follow-up sessions delivered during the supporter activity period. Close consideration was given to the most effective format for all training activities. It was agreed that activities should prioritize smaller group work – which process evaluation data suggested was more effective – and that fewer topics should be covered, but in more depth (with the remaining topics moved to the follow-up sessions). It was also decided that the use of the website and Facebook groups should be more fully integrated into the training (to improve supporter familiarity and confidence with content and process). It was also decided that information and skills training should be integrated across both days, rather than allocated one day each.

Fears and Concerns

Concerns were raised by professional education stakeholders about whether or not the role required too much of students. Fears coalesced around whether PSs would have the requisite maturity to handle potentially inappropriate responses from peers (including online ridicule) and whether or not they could appropriately manage potentially sensitive disclosures, including those raising safeguarding or child protection issues. To signal the responsibility inherent in the role, supporters were asked to sign a 'charter' on completion of the training. This reiterated role expectations and the STASH study values. The training included a session on recognizing and handling sensitive disclosures, with emphasis on swift referral to an appropriate adult if anything gave cause for concern. The researchers emphasized that supporters should not offer any counselling beyond what would typically happen in their everyday friendships.

Sample

The target school was selected from among those expressing interest in participation. It was chosen as typical of schools in the locality (regarding size and relative deprivation). The intervention was implemented over nine weeks, comprising peer nomination, recruitment meetings, supporter training, and five follow-up sessions. Of 163 students in the year group, 31 (19%) were invited to recruitment, having received the highest number of nominations. Of these students, 19 (61% of those invited, 12% of year group) were trained, and 14–17 attended follow-up sessions (attendance varying weekly). No students explicitly withdrew from the PS role, so all 19 students were considered 'completers' and awarded a certificate.

Peer Support Activity

Peer supporters were to establish 'secret' Facebook groups (invitation-only groups with the highest privacy setting), comprising friends and the study trainer. They were encouraged to post messages from the study website to this group and to initiate face-to-face conversations centered on the messages. They were asked to alert friends to the website. Supporters used study cards to advertise a non-sharing version of the website, particularly to students who did not use Facebook. Supporters were supported by a trainer, as well as by an appointed contact teacher. As far as possible, supporters were encouraged to engage with intervention resources flexibly; for instance, they could choose which messages and links to share, and had the option of editing messages into their own words.

Implementation Monitoring

Other studies had used pro forma diaries to track supporter activity, but entries were sometimes fabricated or omitted and did not offer an accurate activity record. In this study, the research team was able to monitor Facebook activity directly, and a decision was made to capture face-to-face conversations via reports to trainers at weekly follow-ups. Regular follow-ups provided an acceptable means of 'checking in', troubleshooting, and encouraging. Interactive learning activities were added to these sessions to maintain interest and momentum. Trainer-led activities include the moderation of group discussions and monitoring posts, supporting the supporters, and facilitating follow-up meetings (weekly or fortnightly) with all PSs for the intervention duration. A further follow-up session conducted evaluation activities.

Participant Acknowledgment

Peer supporters receive formal recognition for their role. Formal academic recognition was provided by a local university certificate and a £10 voucher. Supporters were also given the opportunity to bank time spent on the study toward attainment of a Saltire Award (Scottish Volunteer Award scheme for 12- to 25-year-olds). On a week-to-week basis, commitment was rewarded by a 'Supporter of the Week' prize (a study highlighter).

School Take-Up

Post-pilot student and teacher interviews indicated that the profile of the study across the school was low. Following the suggestion of one supporter, study badges were provided to identify them as such.

REFERENCES

Dodd, S., Widnall, E., Russell, A. E., Curtin, E. L., Simmonds, R., & Limmer, M., et al. (2022). School-based peer education interventions to improve health: A global systematic review of effectiveness. *BMC Public Health, 22,* 2247. https://doi.org/10.1186/s12889-022-14688-3

Fantaye, A. W., Buh, A. W., Idriss-Wheeler, D., Fournier, K., & Yaya, S. (2022). Interventions promoting child sexual and reproductive health and rights in LMICs: A systematic review. *Pediatrics, 149*(s6), e2021053852K SUPPLEMENT. https://doi.org/10.1542/peds.2021-053852K

Farahani, F. K. (2020). Adolescents and young people's sexual and reproductive health in Iran: A conceptual review. *The Journal of Sex Research, 57*(6), 743–780. https://doi.org/10.1080/00224499.2020.1768203

Freestone, J., Siefried, K. J., Prestage, G., Hammoud, M., Molyneux, A., & Bourne, A. (2022). Individual level peer interventions for gay and bisexual men who have sex with men between 2000 and 2020: A scoping review. *PLoS ONE, 17*(7), e0270649. https://doi.org/10.1371/journal.pone.0270649

Kettrey, H. H., Thompson, M. P., Marx, R. A., & Davis, A. J. (2023). Effects of campus sexual assault prevention programs on attitudes and behaviors among American college students: A systematic review and meta-analysis. *Journal of Adolescent Health, 72*(6), 831–844. https://doi.org/10.1016/j.jadohealth.2023.02.022

Kim, C. R., & Free, C. (2008). Recent evaluations of the peer-led approach in adolescent sexual health education: A systematic review. *Perspectives on Sexual and Reproductive Health, 40*(3), 144–151. https://doi.org/10.1363/4014408

Mahat, G., & Scoloveno, M. A. (2018). Effectiveness of adolescent peer education programs on reducing HIV/STI risk: An integrated review. *Research & Theory for Nursing Practice, 32*(2), 168. https://doi.org/10.1891/1541-6577.32.2.168

Mangombe, A., Owiti, P., Madzima, B., Xaba, S., Makoni, T. M., & Takarinda, K. C., et al. (2020). Does peer education go beyond giving reproductive health information? Cohort study in Bulawayo and mount Darwin, Zimbabwe. *BMJ Open, 10,* e034436. https://doi.org/10.1136/bmjopen-2019-034436

Martin, P., Cousin, L., Gottot, S., Bourmaud, A., de La Rochebrochard, E., & Alberti, C. (2020). Participatory interventions for sexual health promotion for adolescents and young adults on the internet: Systematic review. *Journal of Medical Internet Research, 22*(7), e15378. https://doi.org/10.2196/15378

Mitchell, K. R., Purcell, C., Forsyth, R., Barry, S., Hunter, R., & Simpson, S. A., et al. (2020). A peer-led intervention to promote sexual health in secondary schools: The STASH feasibility study. *Public Health Research, 8*(15). https://doi.org/10.3310/phr08150

Newman, P. A., Akkakanjanasupar, A., Tepjan, S., Boborakhimov, S., van Wijngaarden, J. V., & Chonwanarat, N. (2022). Peer Education interventions for HIV prevention and sexual health with young people in mekong region countries: A scoping review and conceptual framework. *Sexual and Reproductive Health Matters, 30*(1), 2129374. https://doi.org/10.1080/26410397.2022.2129374

Niland, R., & Nearchou, F. (2023, January 25). Assessing the effectiveness of school-based sex education in sexual health behaviours: A systematic review. Dublin: University College Dublin. https://doi.org/10.31234/osf.io/g7r8a

O'Farrell, M., Corcoran, P., & Davoren, M. P. (2021). Examining LGBTI + inclusive sexual health education from the perspective of both youth and facilitators: A systematic review. *BMJ Open*, *11*, e047856. https://doi.org/10.1136/bmjopen-2020-047856

Price, N., & Knibbs, S. (2009). How effective is peer education in addressing young people's sexual and reproductive health needs in developing countries? *Children and Society*, *23*(4), 291–302. https://doi.org/10.1111/j.1099-0860.2008.00175.x

Pusmaika, R., & Novianti, L. L. (2017). THE positive impact of school-based peer education program towards adolescent sexual behavior: A systematic review. *LIFE: International Journal of Health and Life-Sciences*, *3(1)*, 69–81. https://doi.org/10.20319/lijhls.2017.31.6981

Siddiqui, M., Kataria, I., Watson, K., & Chandra-Mouli, V. (2020). A systematic review of the evidence on peer education programmes for promoting the sexual and reproductive health of young people in India. *Sexual and Reproductive Health Matters*, *28*(1), 1741494. https://doi.org/10.1080/26410397.2020.1741494

Sun, W. H., Miu, H. Y. H., Wong, C. K. H., Tucker, J. D., & Wong, W. C. W. (2018). Assessing participation and effectiveness of the peer-led approach in youth sexual health education: Systematic review and meta-analysis in more developed countries. *The Journal of Sex Research*, *55*(1), 31–44. https://doi.org/10.1080/00224499.2016.1247779

Tolli, M. V. (2012). Effectiveness of peer education interventions for HIV prevention, adolescent pregnancy prevention and sexual health promotion for young people: A systematic review of European studies. *Health Education Research*, *27*(5), 904–913. https://doi.org/10.1093/her/cys055

United Nations Educational, Scientific and Cultural Organization (2003). *Peer approach in adolescent reproductive health education: Some lessons learned.* Bangkok, Thailand: UNESCO Asia and the Pacific Regional Bureau for Education. ERIC Document Number: ED 478 909SE

Wilson, S. F., Degaiffier, N., Ratcliffe, S. J., & Schreiber, C. A. (2016). Peer Counselling for the promotion of long-acting, reversible contraception among teens: A randomised, controlled trial. *The European Journal of Contraception & Reproductive Health Care*, *21*(5), 380–387. https://doi.org/10.1080/13625187.2016.1214698

Wong, T., Pharr, J. R., Bungum, T., Coughenour, C., & Lough, N. L. (2019). Effects of peer sexual health education on college campuses: A systematic review. *Health Promotion Practice*, *20*(5), 652–666. https://doi.org/10.1177/1524839918794632

Ye, S., Yin, L., Amico, R., Simoni, J., Vermund, S., & Ruan, Y., et al. (2014). Efficacy of peer-led interventions to reduce unprotected anal intercourse among men who have sex with men: A meta-analysis. *PLoS ONE*, *9*(3), e90788. https://doi.org/10.1371/journal.pone.0090788

HIV/AIDS

3

DEFINITION

HIV stands for Human Immunodeficiency Virus. It is a virus that damages the cells in the immune system and weakens the ability to fight everyday infections and diseases. HIV attacks and destroys the infection-fighting CD4 cells (CD4 T lymphocytes) of the immune system. The loss of CD4 cells makes it difficult for the body to fight off infections, illnesses, and certain cancers.

HIV is found in the body fluids of an infected person. This includes semen, vaginal and anal fluids, blood, and breast milk. It is a fragile virus and does not survive outside the body for long. HIV cannot be transmitted through sweat, urine, or saliva. The most common way of getting HIV in the UK is through having anal or vaginal sex without a condom. Other ways of getting HIV include: sharing needles, syringes, or other injecting equipment; transmission from mother to baby during pregnancy, birth, or breastfeeding.

Antiretroviral medicines (or ART) are used to treat HIV. They work by stopping the virus from replicating in the body, allowing the immune system to repair itself, and preventing further damage. HIV is able to develop resistance to a single HIV medicine very easily, but taking a combination of different medicines makes this much less likely. There are effective methods to prevent getting HIV through sex or drug use, including pre-exposure prophylaxis (PrEP) and post-exposure prophylaxis (PEP).

HIV remains a major global public health issue, having claimed an estimated 42.3 million lives to date. There were an estimated 39.9 million people living with HIV at the end of 2023, 65% of whom were in Africa. In 2023, an estimated 630,000 people died from HIV-related causes, and an estimated 1.3 million people acquired HIV.

AIDS stands for Acquired Immune Deficiency Syndrome. The term describes a number of potentially life-threatening infections and illnesses that happen when the immune system has been severely damaged by the HIV.

AIDS occurs at the most advanced stage of infection, which may take many years.

The two are often referred to together as HIV/AIDS. While AIDS cannot be transmitted from one person to another, the HIV can. There is currently no cure for HIV, but there are very effective drug treatments that enable most people with the virus to live a long and healthy life. With an early diagnosis and effective treatments, most people with HIV will not develop any AIDS-related illnesses and will live a near-normal lifespan.

REVIEWS OF EVIDENCE

There were 38 reviews of peer interventions with participants with HIV/AIDS. Fourteen of these (37%) came from or referred to developing countries. This high proportion reflects the concern about HIV/AIDS in developing countries. The earliest reviews also focused on developing countries.

Developing Countries

Van Khoat et al. (2003) reviewed peer education for HIV in Vietnam. Twenty (32%) of Vietnam's 61 provinces and urban areas had functioning peer education programs. Program coordinators of all 20 were interviewed. In addition, on-site reviews were done for half of the 20 programs. A total of 500 peer educators were functioning either independently or as part of one of 79 teams, making an estimated 7,000 total contacts per month with high-risk persons. Despite this, coverage was patchy. Only one province included persons living with HIV/AIDS as peer educators. Six years later, Medley et al. (2009) conducted a more systematic review 1990–2006, including 30 studies. Peer education interventions were significantly associated with increased HIV knowledge (Odds Ratio 2.28), reduced equipment sharing among injection users (OR 0.37) and increased condom use (OR 1.92). There was a nonsignificant effect (but quite a large Odds Ratio) on STI infection (OR 1.22).

A focus on Sub-Saharan Africa characterized the systematic review of Mwale and Muula (2017). The region had the highest burden of HIV, with 70% of HIV infection in general. A systematic review of behavior change interventions targeting adolescents was conducted in seven databases 2000–2015, including 17 studies. There was a dearth of published studies on behavior change, but a number of interventions registered positive outcomes in both knowledge and sexual practices. Peer education stood out as more effective than other psychosocial regimens. Nugroho et al. (2017) investigated behavioral interventions for men who had sex with men and transwomen in Southeast Asia, searching six databases up to 2015, but only five studies met the inclusion criteria. All reported a significant intervention effect on at least one outcome measure (condom use, water-based lubricant use, number of sex partners, HIV prevention knowledge, or willingness to use PrEP).

A narrative review was offered by Azizi et al. (2017) with a focus on adolescents. Six databases were searched from 1991 to 2016, and 53 articles were included. The factors influencing peer education among adolescents were classified as follows: a) characteristics of peer educators (personal, skills, and communication characteristics); b) characteristics of the educational program (theoretical foundations, program transparency, program sustainability, adolescents' comprehensive participation, and evaluation and monitoring; and c) structural characteristics of the educational program (supportive structure, and financial-official structure). Mark et al. (2019) also focused on Sub-Saharan Africa, particularly adolescents. There were few examples of detailed program descriptions describing operational logistics or outcomes around peer support interventions. Nevertheless, these few provided support for the potential utility of peer support to improve outcomes.

Factory workers in low- and middle-income countries were investigated by Chen et al. (2020), searching four databases from 1990 to 2018 and including 13 studies. Intervention improved HIV knowledge, increased condom use, and reduced the use of recreational drugs and alcohol before sex. The detection rate of HIV and other sexually transmitted diseases was increased. Intervention decreased HIV public stigma. Chang et al. (2021) also focused on low and middle-income countries, conducting a rapid review, focused on core journals and reference lists of related reviews. Twenty-nine studies were included. Reported outcomes included reduced HIV incidence and prevalence; increased service access, acceptability and quality; changed risk behaviors; and reduced stigma and discrimination. Contexts of criminalization, under-resourced health systems, and stigma and discrimination influenced these.

Mekong Region countries were investigated by Newman et al. (2022), who conducted a scoping review to identify key characteristics, implementation challenges, and knowledge gaps, especially for adolescents. Seventeen studies were included (from Thailand $n = 7$, Vietnam $n = 5$, Myanmar $n = 3$, Cambodia $n = 1$, and Laos $n = 1$). Focal knowledge gaps emerged in regard to peer educator outcomes (increased knowledge, skill-building, empowerment); interpersonal processes between peer educators and young people (role modeling, social dynamics); and social-structural contexts (sociocultural influences, gendered power relations). Okonkwo et al. (2022) also focused on Sub-Saharan Africa, searching five databases and conducting a systematic review of studies 2008–2020. Empowering patients generally yielded more substantive effects compared to non-adaptive interventions or cash incentives. Motivational counseling and point-of-care CD4 testing seemed most effective. Adolescents in Sub-Saharan Africa were also the focus of Ahmed et al. (2023), who targeted ART adherence and retention in HIV care. Twenty-seven studies were included, encompassing individualized peer support, group-based support, and individualized plus group-based support. Results regarding the efficacy of these interventions were mixed. Although studies evaluating group-based peer support interventions were the most common, most of these studies were not associated with retention, adherence, or mental health outcomes.

Obeagu et al. (2023) focused on behavior change among secondary school adolescents in Uganda. There was a relationship between risk perception and behavior change in HIV/AIDS prevention among high school students. A high proportion of secondary school students thought they were at risk of HIV infection. This perception may be related to having had early sex, being sexually active, or knowing someone has died of HIV. High school students regularly engaged in risky sexual behaviors, such as not using condoms and having multiple partners. However, student behavior was significantly influenced by youth-friendly services and peer education. A systematic review was offered by Shushtari et al. (2023), focusing on adherence to antiretroviral therapy (ART), searching four databases, targeting randomized controlled trials (RCTs), and including 17 studies. There was a significant moderate effect size in the improvement of adherence to ART. Study design, follow-up duration, source of social support, and year of publication significantly moderated effect sizes.

Developed Countries

Maticka-Tyndale and Barnett (2010) focused on youth, evaluating 24 peer-led programs in low- and middle-income countries. These programs demonstrated success in effecting positive change in knowledge and condom use and some success in changing community attitudes and norms. Effects on other sexual behaviors and STI rates were equivocal. Men who had sex with men were addressed by Lorenc et al. (2011) in a systematic review, particularly the uptake of HIV testing. Twenty databases were searched, making this one of the most thorough reviews. Twelve effectiveness studies and one cost-effectiveness study were included. Peer counselling could increase uptake of HIV testing. Findings regarding bundling HIV tests with other tests, peer outreach in community settings, and media campaigns were inconclusive. Behavioral interventions were the interest of Simoni et al. (2011), who included 117 studies. About half were in the developing world and half in Western nations. The majority of studies provided some support for peer interventions according to outcomes such as sexual risk behavior, attitudes and cognitions, HIV knowledge, and substance use. Outcomes assessed using biomarkers and other non-self-report variables were less likely to indicate intervention efficacy.

Milaszewski et al. (2012) focused on older adults, identifying 21 studies on adults aged 50 and over. Three major challenges were ageism in health professionals, older adults' reluctance to discuss sexuality, and their misconception of their HIV risk. Young people in Europe from 1999 to 2010 were the focus of Tolli (2012), who investigated HIV prevention, adolescent pregnancy prevention, and promotion of sexual health. Only five studies were identified. Although a few statistically significant changes were observed, it was concluded that there was no clear evidence of the effectiveness of peer education. Crawford and Bath (2013) investigated people who inject drugs with reference to Hepatitis C virus infection. Peer support models that included opioid substitution treatment had been more common and had been implemented successfully, with a range of outcomes including increased treatment knowledge and uptake and improved service provision.

Factors that maximized success were the focus of Lambert et al. (2013). Between 2008 and 2010, three separate reviews of peer education were undertaken across more than 30 countries in three distinct geographical regions across the globe, seeking to identify determinants of the strengths and weaknesses inherent in approaches to peer education. Several factors were significant contributors to program success, as elements of the social, cultural, political, and organizational context in which peer education was situated. Adherence to a strategy without proper regard to its situational context rarely contributed to effective peer education. Bateganya et al. (2015) were concerned with peer support groups, searching from 1995 to 2014 for the impact of support groups on mortality, morbidity, retention in HIV care, quality of life, and ongoing HIV transmission. Twenty studies were included. Eighteen (90%) of the articles reported largely positive results. Support groups were associated with reduced mortality and morbidity, increased retention in care, and improved quality of life. A meta-analysis was offered by Kanters et al. (2016), who focused on adherence to antiretroviral therapy, searching for RCTs in six electronic databases from 2015 onwards and including 22 trials. They found similar results between global and low- to middle-income (LMIC) settings. Telephone support was superior both globally (Odds Ratio 4.79) and in LMIC settings (OR 4.83). Peer support led to modest improvement in adherence.

Mahat and Scoloveno (2018) searched five databases from 2000 to 2016. Twenty-four quantitative and six qualitative studies were included. There was evidence of the effectiveness of adolescent peer-led HIV education programs on knowledge, attitudes, normative beliefs, and self-efficacy. However, the studies reviewed were equivocal on changes in sexual behavior. The findings of the qualitative/process studies demonstrated perceived program efficacy among staff, peer educators, and learners. A systematic review by Boucher et al. (2020) focused on antiretroviral therapy (ART), searching five databases from 1996 to 2018 and including 13 controlled intervention studies. Findings demonstrated unclear effectiveness for peer-led interventions in ART adherence, but evidence was limited. He et al. (2020) offered a systematic review and meta-analysis, searching four databases and including 60 studies. Peer education was associated with 36% decreased rates of HIV infection among high-risk groups (OR 0.64). Peer education could promote HIV testing (OR 3.19), condom use (OR 2.66), reduced equipment sharing (OR 0.50), and unprotected sex (OR 0.82). Peer education had a consistent effect on behavior change for over 24 months. Peer education was an effective tool with a long-term impact on behavior change.

Behavior change among people who injected drugs was the focus of Mabuie (2020), who searched six relevant journals. Peer education positively influenced norms, attitudes, and beliefs. Ayala et al. (2021) offered a scoping review, searching 1982–2020 for RCTs as well as from quasi-experimental, prospective, pre/post-test evaluation, and cross-sectional study designs. Forty-eight articles were selected. Most studies took place in the global south ($n = 27$), and a third ($n = 17$) involved youth. Sixty-five percent of articles ($n = 31$) described the comparative advantage of peer- and community-led direct services, e.g., prevention and education ($n = 23$); testing, care, and treatment programs ($n = 8$). More than 40 beneficial outcomes were identified, including improved HIV-related knowledge, attitudes, intentions, self-efficacy, risk behaviors, risk appraisals, health literacy, adherence, and viral suppression. Ten studies reported improvements in HIV service access, quality, linkage, utilization, and retention. A systematic review was conducted by Berg et al. (2021), searching eight databases to 2020 and including 20 RCTs from nine different countries. Main outcomes included modest, but superior, retention in care (Risk Ratio 1.07 at 12 months follow-up), antiretroviral therapy adherence (RR 1.06 at 3 months follow-up), and viral suppression (Odds Ratio 6.24 at 6 months follow-up). The evidence for most other main outcomes (ART initiation, CD4 cell count, quality of life, mental health) was promising but too uncertain for firm conclusions.

Costa-Cordella et al. (2022) focused on internet-based peer support interventions, arguing advantages in terms of accessibility and anonymity. Nine studies were included. Internet-based peer support interventions were feasible and acceptable to participants and healthcare workers. Somewhat similarly, Coulson and Buchanan (2022) investigated online peer support groups, searching seven databases and including 22 studies (23% quantitative, 9% mixed methods, and 68% qualitative studies 2007–2019). Engagement with online support groups was empowering for members and could lead to a range of psychosocial benefits (improved self-worth, reduced stigma, improved illness management, and greater confidence in health professionals). Freestone et al. (2022) investigated individual-level peer interventions 2000–2020 for gay and bisexual men, searching five databases and including 38 studies. Four intervention modalities were identified: peer counselling [$n = 6$], groupwork programs [$n = 15$], peer navigation [$n = 7$], and peer education [$n = 10$]. Across intervention modalities, evaluations demonstrated compelling evidence of significant effect.

"Peer navigation" was reviewed by Krulic et al. (2022). Four databases were searched. Six papers drew from RCTs, five from quasi-experimental or pragmatic trials, and four panels, eight qualitative, three mixed methods, and one cross-sectional design were included. Studies primarily reported program effects on continuum of care outcomes. Cabral et al. (2023) offered a scoping review of RCTs, searching four databases from 2017 to 2023 and including 15 studies. The main implementation outcomes presented involved adoption, acceptability, reach, fidelity, feasibility, sustainability, and appropriateness. Positive health impacts included viral suppression of HIV, a significant reduction in systolic blood pressure, and a decrease in the amount of alcohol consumed. Hana et al. (2023) focused on persons living with HIV. Seven databases were searched, and 52 articles were included. The refined theoretical framework presented five areas of peer support, including informational support, instrumental support, emotional support, affiliation support, and appraisal support; including physiological outcomes, psychological outcomes, behavioral outcomes, cognitive outcomes, and social outcomes.

A scoping review by Øgård-Repål et al. (2023) included 53 studies from 2000 to 2021 from 16 countries, but was largely descriptive. Further, focus on interventions addressing secondary prevention as part of a care package was recommended. Zeng et al. (2023) offered an evidence map of peer interventions after searching nine databases for RCTs, nonrandomized controlled trials, and systematic reviews/meta-analyses, finally including 156 studies. There were strengths in the field and a small number of high-quality systematic reviews/meta-analyses showing the effectiveness of interventions. There was a lack of evidence on long-term interventions and follow-ups. A focus on pregnant women and new mothers living with HIV came from Goh et al. (2024), searching seven databases from 1981 to 2022 and including 12 studies. Peer support was perceived to be beneficial in enhancing emotional support among women living with HIV and was well-accepted by them. Peer support played an indispensable role in the lives of women living with HIV and served as a complementary support system to professional and family support.

SINGLE STUDIES

Number of Single Studies

There were 146 single studies of peer interventions with participants with HIV/AIDS. Ninety-six of these (66%) came from or referred to developing countries or disadvantaged groups. As this chapter is so large there is only room to include two single studies.

Exemplar Single Studies Developed Context

The association between peer education, HIV risk perception, and HIV testing uptake was examined, as well as mediated effects (Lin et al., 2021). A cross-sectional survey among 1,188 HIV-uninfected or unknown participants from populations of men who had sex with men (MSM), female sex workers (FSWs), and drug users (DUs) was conducted in seven cities of China. Receiving peer education was associated with higher odds of HIV testing uptake among all of MSM, FSWs, and DUs. Perceiving the risk of HIV infection was associated with higher odds of HIV testing uptake among MSM and DUs. Participants who received peer education tended to be more aware of their risk of HIV infection, which in turn was associated with increased HIV testing uptake among MSM and DUs.

Exemplar Single Studies Developing Context

Rotheram-Borus et al. (2014) conducted an RCT of the efficacy of HIV-positive peer mentors supporting KwaZulu-Natal South African women living with HIV and their infants, from pregnancy through the infant's first year of life. Eight clinics were randomized to receive either standard care or a standard care plus peer mentoring. Peer mentors conducted four antenatal and four postnatal group meetings. At least two post-birth assessment interviews were completed by 57% of women at 1½, 5, 6, or 12 months. Intervention effects were ascertained on 19 measures of maternal and infant wellbeing. Intervention women attended an average of only 4.1 sessions. Nonetheless, significant overall benefits were found for the intervention group compared to the standard care group. Over time, intervention women reported significantly fewer depressive symptoms and fewer underweight infants than comparison women and were significantly more likely to exclusively breastfeed their infants for at least six months. Even though intervention was partial, women benefited from support by HIV-positive peer mentors.

SPECIFIC PROGRAM

The specific program comes from a developing country–South Africa (Atujuna et al., 2021).

Effectiveness

Khuluma is a psychosocial and peer-to-peer intervention that uses text messaging to facilitate support groups for adolescents (15–20-year-olds) living with HIV. Fifty-two adolescents from four clinics in Pretoria and Cape Town were recruited and enrolled to participate in a six-month pilot. Participants were aware of their HIV status, had been on antiretroviral therapy for more than 12 months, and were not suffering from severe depression. Four pre- and post-intervention focus group discussions were conducted with 36 participants. Processes then included engaging participants for minor modifications, forming virtual groups, activating the mHealth platform, and facilitating and delivering the Khuluma intervention. The initial participatory processes helped to tailor the intervention design to participants' needs. The peer-led facilitation of the groups allowed for the provision of sensitive psychosocial support that allowed young people to express themselves freely, develop a sense of self-worth, and interact more. The nature of the mobile technology also allowed participants to build friendships beyond their geographic area and interact with their peers in real-time. The acceptability of the intervention was indicated by follow-up focus group discussions (designed to understand intervention utility, acceptability, and feasibility), conducted in the local language by facilitators fluent in both English and the language spoken in each province. Over-arching themes were social support, stigma and disclosure, medication and adherence, and text message data from 18,253 messages.

Implementation

The Khuluma intervention model was trialed among new mothers in Mexico in 2008, and has been refined, adapted, and replicated in Guatemala (46), the UK, Zimbabwe, Zambia, and South Africa (47), with prior evaluation of the model showing positive health and mental health outcomes for populations experiencing stigma and social isolation (47). The model was adapted in South Africa in 2013, with additional iterations influenced by data obtained from interviews, focus groups, and Khuluma support groups.

Firstly, there was a needs assessment, which included a series of semi-structured individual interviews with health care professionals and 13–18-year-olds to determine challenges associated with treatment uptake, key issues facing young people beyond the clinic, modes of communication and gender norms, and their use of technology. Then young people (some of whom had taken part in Khuluma groups) were engaged in a participatory action research workshop that used artistic methods to create a democratic and "safe space," wherein stakeholders disclosed their personal needs, experiences, and ideas of what they wanted from a support system to facilitators. The discussions identified what forms of support the youth lacked, what kind of support they hoped to get from an intervention, and their acceptance and understanding of using mobile phones to receive support via text messages. The discussions highlighted adolescents' needs around social support, stigma, barriers, facilitators to accessing health care, medical adherence, and mobile technology access and usage. They also elicited insights into recruitment, group facilitation, ideal group sizes, training needs, parental consent, and the adolescent context around school attendance, clinic attendance, and ideal times for session group discussions.

The study was conducted in four adolescent HIV clinics located in Pretoria and Cape Town. The majority of adolescents included in the study had perinatally acquired HIV, came from low socioeconomic backgrounds, and had been receiving HIV care for a number of years. The study population was 52 across the four clinics. Participants were aware of their status, 15–20 years old, and had been on antiretroviral therapy for more than 12 months. Participants were screened for severe depression or other significant mental illness. A sub-sample of the enrolled population was purposively selected and invited to participate in four group discussions. Two of these, comprising seven participants each, were conducted at baseline, while two with 11 participants were conducted 6 months after study enrollment (36 participants in total).

The adapted "Khuluma" intervention (which means "talk/speak" in Zulu) was piloted in 2016, using SMS technology and feature phones. The intervention model was designed to run for three months. Participants were placed in support groups of 8–15 peers who shared experiences of living with HIV. These support groups were virtually enabled through a digital platform, where participants discussed – peer-to-peer, at anytime, anywhere via text message – a range of issues pertinent to their needs. Active facilitation of group sessions occurred Monday to Friday from 3 to 7 p.m. Critically, the model was peer-led, with trained peer mentors facilitating conversations, supported at all times by trained professional counsellors. Participants chose a pseudonym, allowing them to remain anonymous and communicate in small groups. Conversations were externally monitored three times per day by trained staff.

Implementation involved four peer-to-peer support groups of 8–15 participants for 12 weeks, facilitated by a combination of expert professionals and peer mentors. All participants received a new feature phone that had SMS functionality (i.e., not a smart phone) and a registered SIM card to use during the intervention. Participants were given instructions on how to use the phone. Flickswitch©, was the software used to control SIM cards, to distribute and top-up text messages airtime (provided by Vodacom Foundation), and to track usage remotely. Only after enrollment were participants informed they would be allowed to keep the phone at the end of the project. Group SMS messaging was facilitated by a short code that allowed participants to send a message to a central number, from where it would be distributed to their group. This group SMS format was made possible with ZygoHubs© and BulkSMS© technology. ZygoHubs© was a United Kingdom-based group text messaging platform that allowed several individuals to communicate via SMS using a single mobile phone number. ZygoHubs© assigned a mobile phone number to the support group, and all of the messages sent to this designated phone number were delivered to each participant involved in the study via a web interface. BulkSMS©, a South African company, provided the application-to-person messaging service necessary for mobile phones to access ZygoHubs© software. The ZygoHubs© web interface recorded all messages sent to the group mobile phone number from which investigators produced a transcript for analysis. Thus, we were able to provide a confidential SMS messaging system that allowed adolescents to text one another while maintaining anonymity. The system was designed to ensure that third-party access was restricted with access codes only provided to participants, preventing family or friends from accessing messages without the participant's consent. All data were centrally archived.

Participants were asked to decide on personal pseudonyms ("nicknames") (example: Miracle). Beyond the pseudonyms, each participant was allocated a participant ID number, which was used to identify the phone discussion. Four groups were allocated including both males and females, divided by age (two groups of 15–17 years and two of 18–20 years). Over the course of the three-month period, some participants were moved between groups by facilitators dependent on their communication levels and preferences for discussion topics. For example, if a participant was originally put in the group of 15–17-year-olds, but wished to discuss topics of a sexual nature that their peers did not want to discuss, they were moved to the older age group. This meant that the number of participants in each group fluctuated but was never under 8 and never more than 15. In each group, there was a relatively equal mix of participants from Pretoria and Cape Town. Each group was assigned a trained peer mentor to facilitate the conversations.

The professional facilitators consisted of trained counsellors who had implemented the model previously and who had been trained in recruitment, facilitation, and data collection processes. They were tasked with intermittent engagement in all groups, monitoring for problematic behavior or conflict, and identifying participants for referral. The peer mentors were from both provinces, trained via a counsellor-led workshop on group facilitation and use of the technology platform. They were each assigned to one group. The training workshop was adapted from the Positive Connections manual developed for leading information and support groups for adolescents living with HIV. Facilitators were briefed on key issues facing this population, including HIV and AIDS knowledge, adherence to ART, stigma, disclosure, socioeconomic issues, gender-based violence, and education. They were also trained on facilitation skills and techniques such as active listening, empathetic encouragement, non-judgmental communication, asking open-ended questions, validation, and problem solving. They were encouraged to draw on their own experiences as parents, friends, siblings, or caregivers. The facilitators were briefed on the model and technological platform, including troubleshooting and referral processes. The final part of the workshop involved scenario-based thinking, where participants were given difficult issues to engage with and resolve that might occur in the groups, such as conflict between participants, non-participation, suicidal ideation, or a participant spreading a myth. Facilitators were then given a training manual that included the subjects covered in the workshop. This training manual included a curriculum of text messages and suggested responses based on the co-developed list of topics.

Topics in the curriculum were categorized into four areas: (i) HIV knowledge, staying healthy, and treatment adherence; (ii) Growing up, sex and relationships, and sexual health and positive prevention; (iii) Communication and problem solving, personal feelings, and decision-making; (iv) Gender norms, stigma and discrimination, networks, and social support.

Each week, facilitators were given a number of topics to bring up in their groups. Every morning except on weekends, facilitators would check in with the group. Each weekday, after school hours, facilitators would bring up one of these topics. In the first weeks of the intervention, these topics were broadly about getting to know each other, but as the intervention progressed, sensitive topics were discussed. Facilitators were encouraged to follow the lead of participants if they brought up a topic of interest.

REFERENCES

Ahmed, C. V., Doyle, R., Gallagher, D., Imoohi, O., Ofoegbu, U., & Wright, R., et al. (2023). A systematic review of peer support interventions for adolescents living with HIV in sub-Saharan Africa. *AIDS Patient Care and STDs*, *37*(11), 535–559. https://doi.org/10.1089/apc.2023.0094

Atujuna, M., Simpson, N., Ngobeni, M., Monese, T., Giovenco, D., & Pike, C., et al. (2021). Khuluma: Using participatory, peer-led and digital methods to deliver psychosocial support to young people living with HIV in South Africa. *Frontiers in Reproductive Health*, *3*, 687677. https://doi.org/10.3389/frph.2021.687677

Ayala, G., Sprague, L., van der Merwe, L. L., Thomas, R. M., Chang, J., & Arreola, S., et al. (2021). Peer- And community-led responses to HIV: A scoping review. *PLoS ONE 16*(12), e0260555. https://doi.org/10.1371/journal.pone.0260555

Azizi, M., Hamzehgardeshi, Z., & Shahhosseini, Z. (2017). Influential factors for the improvement of peer education in adolescents: A narrative review. *Journal of Pediatrics Review*, *5*(1), e7692. https://doi.org/10.17795/jpr-7692

Bateganya, M., Amanyeiwe, U., Roxo, U., & Dong, M. (2015). The impact of support groups for people living with HIV on clinical outcomes: A systematic review of the literature. *Journal of Acquired Immune Deficiency Syndromes*, *68*(3), S368–S374. https://doi.org/10.1097/QAI.0000000000000519

Berg, R. C., Page, S., & Øgård-Repål, A. (2021). The effectiveness of peer-support for people living with HIV: A systematic review and meta-analysis. *PLoS ONE*, *16*(6), e0252623. https://doi.org/10.1371/journal.pone.0252623

Boucher, L. M., Liddy, C., Mihan, A., & Kendall, C. (2020). Peer-Led self-management interventions and adherence to antiretroviral therapy among people living with HIV: A systematic review. *AIDS and Behavior*, *24*, 998–1022. https://doi.org/10.1007/s10461-019-02690-7

Cabral, J. A., Leite, J. R., Buzinaro, G. S., Leite, H. Q., & Bomfim, R. A. (2023). Peer Support implementation strategy in the primary health care setting: Scoping review. *Acta Paulista De Enfermagem*, *36*, eAPESPE023333. https://doi.org/10.37689/acta-ape/2023ARSPE023333

Chang, J., Shelly, S., Busz, M., Stoicescu, C., Iryawan, A. R., & Madybaeva, D., et al. (2021). Peer driven or driven peers? A rapid review of Peer involvement of people who use drugs in HIV and harm reduction services in low and middle-income countries. *Harm Reduction Journal*, *18*, 15. https://doi.org/10.1186/s12954-021-00461-z

Chen, D. H., Luo, G. F., Meng, X. J., Wang, Z. X., Cao, B. L., & Yuan, T. W., et al. (2020). Efficacy of HIV interventions among factory workers in low- and middle-income countries: A systematic review. *BMC Public Health*, *20*(1), 1310. https://doi.org/10.1186/s12889-020-09333-w

Costa-Cordella, S., Grasso-Cladera, A., Rossi, A., Duarte, J., Guiñazu, F., & Cortes, C. P. (2022). Internet-based peer support interventions for people living with HIV: A scoping review. *PLOS One*, *17*(8), e0269332. https://doi.org/10.1371/journal.pone.0269332

Coulson, N. S., & Buchanan, H. (2022). The role of online support groups in helping individuals affected by HIV and AIDS: Scoping review of the literature. *Journal of Medical Internet Research*, *24*(7), e27648. https://doi.org/10.2196/27648

Crawford, S., & Bath, N. (2013). Peer Support models for people with a history of injecting drug use undertaking assessment and treatment for hepatitis c virus infection. *Clinical Infectious Diseases*, *57*(S2), S75–9. https://doi.org/10.1093/cid/cit297

Freestone, J., Siefried, K. J., Prestage, G., Hammoud, M., Molyneux, A., & Bourne, A. (2022). Individual level peer interventions for gay and bisexual men who have sex with men between 2000 and 2020: A scoping review. *PLoS ONE*, *17*(7), e0270649. https://doi.org/10.1371/journal.pone.0270649

Goh, H. Q., Nelson, L. E., Teo, W. Z., Aidoo-Frimpong, G., Ramos, S. R., & Shorey, S. (2024). Perspectives and thoughts of pregnant women and new mothers living with HIV receiving peer support: A mixed studies systematic review. *Journal of Advanced Nursing*, *80*(7), 2715–2727. https://doi.org/10.1111/jan.16014

Hana, S., Zhang, Y. Z., Yang, X. X., Chai, X. R., Guo, J. Z., & Zhang, L., et al. (2023). The effectiveness and sustainability of peer support interventions for two persons living with HIV: A realist synthesis. *BMJ Global Health*, *8*(2), e010966. https://doi.org/10.1136/bmjgh-2022-010966

He, J., Wang, Y., Du, Z., Liao, J., He, N., & Hao, Y. T. (2020). Peer Education for HIV prevention among high-risk groups: A systematic review and meta-analysis. *BMC Infectious Diseases*, *20*, 338. https://doi.org/10.1186/s12879-020-05003-9

Kanters, S., Park, J. J. H., Chan, K., Ford, N., Forrest, J., & Thorlund, K., et al. (2016). Use of peers to improve adherence to antiretroviral therapy: A global network meta-analysis. *Journal of the International AIDS Society*, *19*, 21141. http://dx.doi.org/10.7448/IAS.19.1.21141

Krulic, T., Brown, G., & Bourne, A. (2022). A scoping review of peer navigation programs for people living with HIV: Form, function and effects. *AIDS and Behavior*, *26*, 4034–4054. https://doi.org/10.1007/s10461-022-03729-y

Lambert, S. M., Debattista, J., Bodiroza, A., Martin, J., Staunton, S., & Walker, R. (2013). Effective peer education in HIV: Defining factors that maximise success. *Sexual Health*, *10*(4), 325–331. https://doi.org/10.1071/SH12195

Lin, Y. X., Li, C. X., Wang, L., Jiao, K., & Ma, W. (2021). The mediated effect of HIV risk perception in the relationship between peer education and HIV testing uptake among three key populations in China. *AIDS Research and Therapy*, *18*(8). https://doi.org/10.1186/s12981-021-00334-2

Lorenc, T., Marrero-Guillamón, I., Aggleton, P., Cooper, C., Llewellyn, A., & Lehmann, A., et al. (2011). Promoting the uptake of HIV testing among men who have sex with men (MSM): Systematic review of effectiveness and cost-effectiveness. *Sexually Transmitted Infections*, *87*(4), 272–278. https://doi.org/10.1136/sti.2010.048280

Mabuie, M. A. (2020). Role of peer educators in behaviour change communication interventions for HIV prevention among people who inject drugs: Systematic review article. *Technium Social Sciences Journal*, *10*, 189–200.

Mahat, G., & Scoloveno, M. A. (2018). Effectiveness of adolescent peer education programs on reducing HIV/STI risk: An integrated review. *Research and Theory for Nursing Practice*, *32*(2). https://doi.org/10.1891/1541-6577.32.2.168

Mark, D., Hrapcak, S., Ameyan, W., Lovich, R., Ronan, A., & Schmitz, K., et al. (2019). Peer Support for adolescents and young people living with HIV in sub-Saharan Africa: Emerging insights and a methodological agenda. *Current HIV/AIDS Reports*, *16*(6), 467–474. https://doi.org/10.1007/s11904-019-00470-5

Maticka-Tyndale, E., & Barnett, J. P. (2010). Peer-led interventions to reduce HIV risk of youth: A review. *Evaluation and Program Planning*, *33*(2), 98–112. https://doi.org/10.1016/j.evalprogplan.2009.07.001

Medley, A., Kennedy, C., O'Reilly, K., & Sweat, M. (2009). Effectiveness of peer education interventions for HIV prevention in developing countries: A systematic review and meta-analysis. *AIDS Education and Prevention*, *21*(3), 181–206. https://doi.org/10.1521/aeap.2009.21.3.181

Milaszewski, D., Greto, E., Klochkov, T., & Fuller–Thomson, E. (2012). A systematic review of education for the prevention of HIV/AIDS among older adults. *Journal of Evidence-Based Social Work*, *9*(3), 213–230. https://doi.org/10.1080/15433714.2010.494979

Mwale, M., & Muula, A. S. (2017). Systematic review: A review of adolescent behavior change interventions [BCI] and their effectiveness in HIV and AIDS prevention in sub-Saharan Africa. *BMC Public Health*, *17*, 718. https://doi.org/10.1186/s12889-017-4729-2

Newman, P. A., Akkakanjanasupar, P., Tepjan, S., Boborakhimov, S., & van Wijngaarden, J. W. V., et al. (2022). Peer Education interventions for HIV prevention and sexual health with young people in Mekong region countries: A scoping review and conceptual framework. *Sexual and Reproductive Health Matters*, *30*(1), 2129374. https://doi.org/10.1080/26410397.2022.2129374

Nugroho, A., Erasmus, V., Zomer, T. P., Wu, Q., & Richardus, J. H. (2017). Behavioral interventions to reduce HIV risk behavior for MSM and transwomen in southeast Asia: A systematic review. *Aids Care - Psychological and Socio-Medical Aspects of AIDS/HIV*, *29*(1), 98–104. https://doi.org/10.1080/09540121.2016.1200713

Obeagu, E. I., Obeagu, G. U., Ede, M. O., Odo, E. O., & Buhari, H. A. (2023). Translation of HIV/AIDS knowledge into behavior change among secondary school adolescents in Uganda: A review. *Medicine*, *102*(49), e36599. https://doi.org/10.1097/MD.0000000000036599

Øgård-Repål, A., Berg, R. C., & Fossum, M. (2023). Peer Support for people living with HIV: A scoping review. *Health Promotion Practice*, *24*(1), 172–190. https://doi.org/10.1177/15248399211049824

Okonkwo, N. E., Blum, A., Viswasam, N., Hahn, E., Ryan, S., & Turpin, G., et al. (2022). A systematic review of linkage-to-care and antiretroviral initiation implementation strategies in low- and middle-income countries across sub-saharan Africa. *AIDS and Behavior, 26*(7), 2123–2134. https://doi.org/10.1007/s10461-021-03558-5

Rotheram-Borus, M. J., Richter, L. M., van Heerden, A., van Rooyen, H., Tomlinson, M., & Harwood, J. M., et al. (2014). A cluster randomized controlled trial evaluating the efficacy of peer mentors to support South African women living with HIV and their infants. *PLoS ONE, 9*(1), e84867. https://doi.org/10.1371/journal.pone.0084867

Shushtari, Z. J., Salimi, Y., Sajjadi, H., & Paykani, T. (2023). Effect of social support interventions on adherence to antiretroviral therapy among people living with HIV: A systematic review and meta-analysis. *AIDS and Behavior, 27*(5), 1619–1635. https://doi.org/10.1007/s10461-022-03894-0

Simoni, J. M., Nelson, K. M., Franks, J. C., Yard, S. S., & Lehavot, K. (2011). Are peer interventions for HIV efficacious? A systematic review. *AIDS and Behavior, 15*(8), 1589–1595. https://doi.org/10.1007/s10461-011-9963-5

Tolli, M. V. (2012). Effectiveness of peer education interventions for HIV prevention, adolescent pregnancy prevention and sexual health promotion for young people: A systematic review of European studies. *Health Education Research, 27*(5), 904–913. ERIC Number: EJ979730

Van Khoat, D., West, G. R., Valdiserri, R. O., & Phan, N. T. (2003). Peer Education for HIV prevention in the socialist Republic of Vietnam: A national assessment. *Journal of Community Health, 28*(1), 1–17. https://doi.org/10.1023/A:1021321704417

Zeng, Y., Wan, B., Zhao, X., Xie, P., Yang, W. L., & Yan, X., et al. (2023). HIV peer education interventions: An evidence map. *Research Square.* https://doi.org/10.21203/rs.3.rs-3176735/v1

Cancer

4

DEFINITION

Cancer is a condition where cells in a specific part of the body grow and reproduce uncontrollably. Such neoplasms can be benign or malignant (cancerous). Cancerous cells invade and destroy surrounding healthy tissue. Cancer often begins in one part of the body before spreading to other areas (metastasis). The four most common types of cancer are breast cancer, lung cancer, prostate cancer, and bowel cancer, but there are more than 200 different types of cancer. The chance of survival depends on the type of cancer and extent of the disease at the start of treatment. Many cancers occur more commonly in developed countries, and survival is worse, partly because the types of cancer that are most common there are harder to treat than those associated with developed countries. The risk of suicide in people with cancer is approximately double. Breastfeeding is associated with reduced mortality in children aged less than five years. The studies below are categorized into the preventive and the corrective (about patients who already had cancer).

REVIEWS OF EVIDENCE

There were 29 reviews of research literature on peer education/counselling/support for cancer. Ten of these dealt with specific kinds of cancer, including many of the most common kinds. Interestingly, there was no corrective review of lung cancer, although Chapter 10 in this book deals with smoking, the major cause of lung cancer. Fourteen reviews concerned all types of cancer, which might have resulted in some confounding between different responses to different types, and of course, the quality of studies tended to improve as the years passed. Further studies focused on digital corrective

DOI: 10.1201/9781003438366-4

peer support (three studies), the role of physical activity in cancer, and peer supporters rather than the supported.

Breast Cancer–Preventive

Two reviews concerned preventive peer education/counselling/support for cancer. Shakya et al. (2017) searched six databases and selected 47 randomized controlled trials (RCTs) and quasi-experimental studies. In low- and middle-income countries, peer support significantly increased exclusive breastfeeding at three months compared to usual care, and at three months and at six months. Peer support also increased the initiation of breastfeeding within the first hour of life and decreased pre-lacteal feeding. In high-income countries, peer support only increased exclusive breastfeeding at 3 months. This study is also reported in Chapter 12 on breastfeeding.

Breast and cervical cancer screening uptake among women in rural communities was the focus of Atere-Roberts et al. (2020). Only Medline was used, and eight studies only from the USA from 2006 to 2019 were included. Interventions focused on uptake of initial screening rather than repeated screening. Study populations comprised multiple racial/ethnic groups. Of these eight studies, six increased post-intervention screening uptakes in rural communities. Some interventions used native language materials and found improved effectiveness.

Breast Cancer–Corrective

D'Egidio et al. (2017) searched two databases up to 2016 and included 35 articles, including 24 RCTs. Peer counselling included lifestyle counseling, physical activity, and nutritional counseling. Exercise counseling was effective to improve shoulder mobility, healing wounds, and limb strength. All the analyzed studies indicated favorable results for interventions. Pefbrianti et al. (2018) investigated the effect of peer education in improving quality of life and knowledge. Four databases were searched from 2006 to 2016, and ten articles were included. All studies showed significant improvements. Seven databases were searched by Hu et al. (2019), including 15 RCT studies. Overall, there were more positive effects than invalid or negative effects across peer interventions. Peer education showed promising effects on stress management, quality of life, and healthy behaviors. Web-based group peer support without peer training was not effective, however.

Tan et al. (2023) conducted a systematic review and meta-analysis of RCTs for breast cancer patients, searching eight databases to 2021 and including 14 studies. Peer support significantly improved quality of life (effect size = 0.69) and anxiety (effect size = 0.45). Peer support interventions effectively improved psychosocial adaptation in breast cancer patients.

Bowel Cancer

A meta-analysis by Hu et al. (2020) investigated colorectal cancer screening in ethnic minorities. Six databases were searched for RCTs, and 13 studies were included. Results showed peer support could raise awareness and intention to undergo the screening and also increase actual screening implementation more significantly than usual care. Results were stronger with Asian Americans. However, church-based programs require enhanced management to maintain their fidelity.

Prostate Cancer

Pyle et al. (2021) conducted a scoping review of online prostate cancer communities. Four databases were searched and 21 studies were included. Some studies were quite elderly. Men reported that sharing information helped them deal with their diagnosis and treatment side effects. They also gained a sense of camaraderie with men who shared similar experiences.

Blood Cancer

Peer support among patients with hematologic malignancies and/or patients who had undergone hematopoietic stem cell transplantation was investigated by Amonoo et al. (2022). Five databases were searched, and eight studies were included. Four studies highlighted the benefits of peer support, such as improved physical symptoms.

Head and Neck Cancer

Hatton et al. (2022) conducted a scoping review on quality-of-life impacts in head and neck cancer. Five databases were used between 1981 and 2020, and ten papers were included. Five were qualitative, two cross-sectional, one case-control, one cohort, and one quasi-experimental. All papers agreed that peer-to-peer support could be beneficial in terms of sharing information, gaining an insight into the future, and connecting with others, helping to reduce the feeling of uncertainty and isolation. Those who engaged in peer support as mentors reported feeling important and valuable.

Cancer Overall

Papers which reviewed outcomes of peer education/counseling/support for all types of cancer will be discussed in chronological order. An early paper by Dunn et al. (2003) selected 25 articles, suggesting that peer support programs helped by providing emotional and informational support from the perspective of shared personal experience. However, a paucity of RCTs was noted. This might stem from inherent difficulties in studying what was essentially a naturalistically occurring interpersonal dynamic in complex social and community contexts. Campbell et al. (2004) conducted a systematic literature review of studies from 1983 to 2003, including 17 papers. Most lacked a theoretical framework, adequate program descriptions, data on non-participants, and validated instruments. However, consistent informational, emotional, and instrumental benefits were identified. A focus on psychosocial adjustment led to a search of three databases from 1980 to 2007 (Hoey et al., 2008), including 43 articles, ten of which were RCTs. Five models of peer support were identified: 1–1 face-to-face, 1–1 telephone, group face-to-face, group telephone, and group Internet. Papers indicated a high level of satisfaction with peer-support programs; however, evidence for psychosocial benefit was mixed. One-on-one face-to-face and group Internet peer-support programs appeared the most effective.

Also in 2008, Macvean et al. searched three databases to 2007 reporting one-to-one support programs using volunteers, including 28 articles. Nineteen (69%) reported peer-support programs, with 12 of these describing peer-support programs for women with breast cancer. Four were RCTs. Most papers reported that programs were beneficial. Meyer et al. (2015) also focused on one-to-one peer support, searching two databases from 2007 to 2014 and including 13 studies (with four RCTs). All studies reported high participant satisfaction with peer support, and the majority noted positive outcomes regarding psychological adjustment. A meta-analysis by Lee and Suh (2018) searched six databases from 1997 to –2017 and included 18 studies including 16 RCTs. While many outcomes were positive, an additional tiered evaluation of higher quality was needed.

Walshe and Roberts (2018) offered a scoping review of peer support for patients with advanced cancer, reviewing 22 articles describing three forms of peer support (one-to-one, group, and online), reaching primarily those who were women, middle-aged, and well educated. Peer support was likely to be beneficial. Three databases were searched from 2014 to 2016 in a scoping review by Kowitt et al. (2019), including the most recent 100 articles, of which 80% were in the USA and 26% were RCTs. A number of studies focused on breast cancer (32%) or multiple cancer sites (23%). Only 2% targeted end-of-life care. Interventions were primarily phone-based (44%) or delivered in a clinic setting (44%). Peer Support appeared to be widely used across the cancer care continuum but outcomes were not well summarized. Boghosian et al. (2021) focused on women with a BRCA1 or BRCA2 gene mutation, likely to increase the risk of heredi-tary breast and ovarian cancers. In a scoping review, four databases were searched and 23 articles included, suggesting that telephone-based peer-to-peer counselling and online communities improved patient knowledge and psychosocial functioning and could overcome challenges such as scheduling and travel, but may have other challenges with recruitment and retaining of participants. Overall, all the forms of intervention were well-received by participants; and some reduced distress, depression, and anxiety.

Describing cancer peer support programs in "real world" settings was the aim of Brodar et al. (2022), who identified 100 programs; half were invited to participate in semi-structured interviews and 29 agreed. The researchers observed eight primary themes. Allocating time and effort to recruit, train, track and retain peer supporters was a constant challenge. Solutions included recruiting previous recipients to become peer supporters or incorporating them as paid staff. All programs mentioned the importance of ongoing support and backup for the supporters. Jablotschkin et al. (2022) reviewed qualitative studies, focusing on face-to-face community support groups. Three databases were searched from 2000 to 2022 and 20 studies were included. All studies indicated that participation in a peer-led group led to multiple perceived ben-efits: informational support, shared experience, learning from others, helping others as well as cultivating humor as a coping strategy. Challenges included: confrontation with the suffering of others, divergent information needs, dis-tressing group dynamics, and leadership and sustainability.

The effects of peer support interventions on quality of life, depression, anxiety and self-efficacy were reviewed by Zhang et al. (2022). Seven data-bases were searched in 2020 and 17 studies were included. Meta-analysis indicated significant beneficial effects of peer support on quality-of-life (effect size = 0.48), depression (effect size = 0.23), anxiety (effect size = 0.24), and self-efficacy (effect size = 0.22). Peer support delivered in the mixed mode (face-to-face plus telephone) contributed more than peer sup-port delivered in the single mode. Clougher et al. (2023) explored quali-tative evidence, searching until mid-2023 and including 11 articles. Four core areas were identified; peer support could: create understanding and a mutual therapeutic and emotional connection; facilitate an educational and supportive patient-centered journey; should monitor group members for unpleasant emotional experiences; and have professional supervision of recruitment and training.

Eighteen RCTs on peer-to-peer support from 2000 to early 2023 were reviewed by Kiemen et al. (2023). Main settings were dyadic support via telephone, face-to-face (FTF), and web-based online support. Beneficial effects were apparent in FTF settings and quality-of-life outcomes, but there were only small effects on depression/anxiety, coping or sexual functioning. Vrontaras et al. (2023) focused on post-traumatic growth in cancer – positive psychological change experienced as a result of struggling with highly challenging and stressful life circumstances. The authors searched five databases from 1994 onward and located 37 trials (46 articles with sample size ≥ 30), 42% RCTs. Participants were mainly female (83%) with a single cancer type (54%). Peer support and health coaching interventions were effective in producing post-traumatic growth (effect size = 0.28).

Digital Support

Some of the preceding reviews have incorporated mention of online peer support as well as other modalities, but two reviews focused on only this area. Ihrig et al. (2020) examined online peer-to-peer support specifically for prostate cancer patients, including 24 studies, mostly descriptive. Online support groups played a significant role in patients' treatment decision-making and social environment. Information exchange was predominant, but emotional and supportive content was also important. Allison et al. (2021), searched five databases and included 41 articles. Online spaces provided more accessible opportunities for peer support, given the medical and logistical restrictions on FTF interaction associated with cancer and treatment. Just 12 studies required users to meet a minimum frequency of posting, posting or reading, or otherwise accessing the online community. Quantitative results for depression and anxiety were mixed, and appeared to depend on how individuals engaged and interacted. Qualitative findings suggested clear value in connecting and sharing experiences with those in similar situations, benefits which might not be well captured quantitatively.

Physical Activity

The impact of physical activity interventions on cancer patients was investigated by Smith-Turchyn et al. (2023), Six databases were searched up to 2022 and 12 articles were included, on six activity interventions. Most interventions

(83%) had peers operating on a one-to-one basis. All articles demonstrated that peer support led to significantly higher levels of physical activity.

Peer Supporters

Que et al. (2023) reviewed the experiences of peer *supporters*, noting that many cancer survivors were first supported then became supporters. Seven databases were searched and ten articles were included, from which 29 themes were distilled, grouped into benefits and challenges. Peer supporters gained social support, growth, and recovery, but also experienced various challenges.

SINGLE STUDIES

Number of Single Studies

There were 100 single studies of peer education/counselling/support for cancer. Thirty-three of these (33%) explored preventive approaches, while 67 focused on corrective measures. For preventive studies, 10 out of 33 (30%) focused on developing countries and 23 on developed countries. For corrective studies, 10 out of 67 (15%) focused on developing countries and 57 on developed countries. While for preventive studies the proportion of studies focused on developing countries was similar to that for other medical conditions (e.g., Diabetes, Chapter 5), for corrective studies this proportion was much lower. Thus, developing countries did not have as many corrective studies as developed countries. Frequently occurring cancers such as breast cancer and prostate cancer tended to attract a greater number of studies. Given the number of reviews was so large, only four single studies will be featured below. One preventive and one corrective study will be described for each context (developed or developing country).

Exemplar Single Studies Developed Context

The aim of the quasi-experimental study of Alp Dal et al. (2022) was to raise awareness of gynecological cancers in university students via peer education and lead to behavioral changes to that effect. Ten peer educators reached

90 university students. One week prior to the program, the peer educators administered a questionnaire which assessed behavioral changes along with the Gynecologic Cancer Awareness Scale (GCAS). Peer educators re-administered the questionnaire one week after the peer education, and then again one month later. The average score of the students who received training from peer educators was 151 before the education, 181 after one week of peer education, and 179 after one month, a highly statistically significant difference. Participants sustained their enhanced knowledge and reported behavioral changes.

The objective of Walshe et al. (2019) was to determine the feasibility of delivering and investigating a novel peer mentor intervention to promote and maintain psychological well-being in people with advanced cancer. A controlled trial of intervention plus usual care, vs. usual care alone was coupled with a qualitative process evaluation. Quantitative data assessed the quality of life, coping styles, depression, social support, and use of healthcare and other supports. Qualitative interviews probed participant experiences. Twelve peer mentors worked with 12 patients (from 181 eligible). Those in the intervention group experienced an improvement in quality of life and those in the control group a decline in most domains. Pragmatic trials, where the effectiveness of an intervention is tested in real-world routine practice, may be more appropriate than other forms of research.

Exemplar Single Studies Developing Context

Sadoh et al. (2021) noted that early breast cancer detection strategies such as mammography were beyond the reach of most women in sub-Saharan Africa, partly because of lack of awareness and late presentation. This study investigated the effect of peer education to create awareness about breast cancer and breast self-examination among in-school female adolescents of four secondary schools in Benin City, Nigeria. Knowledge about breast cancer and breast self-examination were assessed by questionnaire in about 30% of each school population. Then 124 students were selected from the schools (one student per class) as peer trainers, to provide training for their classmates. After two weeks knowledge was reassessed. There were 1337 and 1201 students who responded to the pre- and post-training questionnaires respectively. The mean breast cancer knowledge score (21) prior to training was low and it statistically significantly improved to 56 following training ($p < 0.0001$). Before peer training 906 (68%) students knew about breast self-examination, while after significantly more students (1,134, 95%) knew.

A study was conducted in Myanmar to evaluate the effect of a peer support intervention on quality of life in breast cancer patients (Naung et al.,

2021). A total of 74 patients were randomly assigned to a peer support during chemotherapy or a control group. Quality of Life was assessed using the European Organisation for Research and Treatment of Cancer Quality of Life Questionnaire. There was no significant difference in pre-test between the intervention and control groups in socio-demographic characteristics, medical history, global health status/quality-of-life, physical, emotional, cognitive, and social functioning. At post-test, the intervention group had significantly higher mean scores on global health status/quality-of-life ($p = 0.017$), physical functioning ($p < 0.001$), role functioning ($p < 0.001$), emotional functioning ($p < 0.001$), cognitive functioning ($p = 0.002$) and social functioning ($p = 0.002$), and significantly lower mean scores on fatigue ($p = 0.009$) and nausea/vomiting ($p = 0.022$) than the control group.

SPECIFIC PROGRAM

The specific program is of a corrective intervention from a developed country (Allicock et al., 2017). It concerns Peer Connect, a program for African American breast cancer survivors and their caregivers, which adopted a train-the-trainer approach. Breast cancer survival inequities persist for African American women, who experience only 79% 5-year survival rates compared to 91% for white women. Compared to white survivors, African American breast cancer survivors are more likely to die from comorbid conditions. The research team ($n = 2$) trained the Community Coaches ($n = 5$, volunteer cancer survivors and caregivers) who trained the breast cancer survivors and caregivers as Guides ($N = 9$), who then trained the cancer survivors and caregivers in the community (Partners).

Effectiveness

The Community Coaches initially relied heavily on advice giving but improved to use other strategies (e.g., asking open questions). Three of the five Community Coaches then conducted the three-day training for nine Guides. They had some difficulty providing examples of personal reflections. However, by the end of Day 2, the Community Coaches seemed more comfortable and confident. They adhered closely to most of the protocols, except for the Reflections and Using Values sessions, where some of the group activities were shortened or skipped due to the lack of time. Protocol adherence was roughly 85%.

Of the five Community Coaches, four had ratings that showed competence; none met the criteria for reflections to questions ratio or open questions; but all displayed competency in relevant skills. Of the nine Guides, five met the criteria for competency; none met the criteria for reflections to questions ratio; four were at least proficient in using open questions; and two scored at competency. At pre-test, one Community Coach and two Guides provided an appropriate response (e.g., used reflections and/or asked open questions) to either scenario. At post-test, all Community Coaches and seven of the nine Guides provided an appropriate response to the first scenario, and all Guides provided an appropriate response to the subsequent scenario.

In general, both Community Coaches and Guides felt that the training provided concrete skills to help them communicate more effectively with potential Partners, was empowering, and the training sequence flowed well. Both groups said that using open questions and summarizing were the most challenging communication skills. Perceived self-efficacy to use the skills was rated on a 10-point scale. Mean self-efficacy for Community Coaches at pre-test was 5.3 and at post-test was 7.4. For Guides scores were 6.1 at pre-test and post-test 9.1.

Implementation

Guides were trained using the Peer Connect DVD and manual and matched to Partners. The focus was patient-centered: listening, reflecting and avoiding unsolicited advice. Guides were trained in communication skills: asking open-ended questions, reflective listening, building motivation (importance, confidence, and values clarification), moving toward change (overcoming barriers and matching resources with participant interests), summarizing, and goal setting. The manual included program description, roles and responsibilities, evaluation tools, and additional resources for program implementation. A Coordinator's manual provided detailed guidance to aid in program implementation.

Guide and Partner pairings were based on participant type (survivor or caregiver), gender, and race when possible. All conversations between Guides and Partners were initiated over the telephone, but could be extended to FTF conversations. The Community Coaches lived in the local community and could better connect to breast cancer survivors and caregivers than outside researchers, and the new training knowledge could add to local capacity. Partner organizations recruited and trained Guides. They used flyers, word-of-mouth and emails to existing cancer-related listservs to recruit African American breast cancer survivors and caregivers.

Guides who signed up to be trained by Community Coaches attended the three-day training workshop and signed on to attend monthly 90-min supplemental sessions (Guide Gatherings) for 6 months to reinforce skills, gain additional practice, and problem-solve issues. They agreed to participate as a Guide for a year. Community Coaches were also expected to attend Guide Gatherings and serve for one year. Eligibility criteria for Community Coaches and Guides were that they be over 18 years old, English-speaking, and either a breast cancer survivor (at least one year post-treatment) or experienced in caregiving for someone diagnosed with cancer. Financial rewards ($100/day for each training day) were provided to Community Coaches and Guides at training completion.

Participants practiced approaches for communicating with and supporting Partners' needs using individual, dyadic, and group reflective exercises, discussion and shared problem-solving, interactive skill sessions and writing exercises. The training also included maintaining confidentiality and boundaries of providing peer support. The training did not have a specific behavioral focus, e.g., getting more physical activity or communicating to a health provider about fear of cancer recurrence. The program's intent was to be able to meet Partners where they were with whatever issue they brought to the Guides.

Day 1 included an Introduction/program overview, how Peer Connect worked, providing support and maintaining confidentiality, the DVD Part I: Communication Skills: Open Questions, Reflective Listening, and use of affirmations. Day 2 included a review of day 1, building motivation: values, importance and confidence, summarizing, and using the skills in a full conversation. Day 3 included a review of day 2, DVD Part II: A first conversation with partners, sharing resources and other information, making a referral for counseling, handling requests for medical/other advice, setting up the next call and continuing the partnership.

Both Community Coaches and Guides completed a 15–20-minute practice phone counseling conversation via telephone with a research team member one week after the conclusion of their training. A member of the research team role-played as a breast cancer survivor or caregiver. All practice conversations were recorded and Community Coaches and Guides received immediate verbal feedback from the research team members. The recordings were coded. Global ratings included two components: one to capture counselor empathy (i.e., the extent to which the interviewer understood and/or made an effort to grasp the Partner's perspective) and the second for spirit (i.e., the overall competence of the interviewer in using evocation, collaboration, and autonomy), each rated from 1 to 5, with higher scores indicating higher success. The second domain, behavioral counts, tallied four specific behaviors: (1) reflection to question ratio; (2) percent open-ended questions; (3) percent complex questions; and (4) percentage adherent or non-adherent statements. Second, both Community Guides and Coaches responded in writing to two fictitious scenarios regarding a potential, topic-relevant conversation.

To assess acceptability three approaches were used. First, at pre- and post-test, to evaluate the utility of the training, the researchers assessed trainee perceived self-efficacy (0 = not all – 10 = very much). Second, at post-test, they inquired about usefulness of the training (0 = not all – 10 = very much); both used a 5-point Likert scale: strongly agree to strongly disagree. Finally, a facilitated discussion (debriefing) allowed participants to feedback regarding the training format and content, their perceptions of their readiness to use the skills, and any training needs they felt had gone unmet.

The researchers also built in formal monthly program support calls to assist community partners with any program issues or feedback as needed. Given the modest success in learning the skills, more technical support for Community Coaches was needed. For example, they could conduct a mock training and get feedback and additional training tips from the research team prior to the actual program start.

REFERENCES

Allicock, M., Haynes-Maslow, L., Johnson, L., Carpenter, W. R., Vines, A. I., & Belle, D. G., et al. (2017). Peer connect for African American breast cancer survivors and caregivers: A train-the-trainer approach for peer support. *Translational Behavioral Medicine*, 7(3), 495–505. https://doi.org/10.1007/s13142-017-0490-4

Allison, K. R., Patterson, P., Guilbert, D., Noke, M., & Husson, O. (2021). Logging on, reaching out, and getting by: A review of self-reported psychosocial impacts of online peer support for people impacted by cancer. In *Proceedings of the ACM on Human-Computer Interaction*, 5, CSCW1, Article 95. https://doi.org/10.1145/3449169

Alp Dal, N., Tuna, A., & Yavuz, T. (2022). Is peer education effective in raising awareness of gynecological cancers? *The Journal of International Education Science*, 30, 47–57. https://doi.org/10.29228/INESJOURNAL.54986

Amonoo, H. L., Harnedy, L. E., Staton, S. C., Longley, R. M., Daskalakis, E., & El-Jawahri, A., et al. (2022). Peer support in patients with hematologic malignancies: A systematic review. *Bone Marrow Transplantation*, 57(8), 1240–1249. https://doi.org/10.1038/s41409-022-01709-3

Atere-Roberts, J., Smith, J. L., & Hall, I. J. (2020). Interventions to increase breast and cervical cancer screening uptake among rural women: A scoping review. *Cancer Causes Control*, *31*(11), 965–977. https://doi.org/10.1007/s10552-020-01340-x

Boghosian, T., McCuaig, J. M., Carlsson, L., & Metcalfe, K. A. (2021). Psychosocial interventions for women with a BRCA1 or BRCA2 mutation: A scoping review. *Cancers*, *13*, 1486. https://doi.org/10.3390/cancers13071486

Brodar, K. E., Carlisle, V., Tang, P. Y., & Fisher, E. B. (2022). Identification and characterization of peer support for cancer prevention and care: A practice review. *Journal of Cancer Education*, *37*, 645–654. https://doi.org/10.1007/s13187-020-01861-8

Campbell, H. S., Phaneuf, M. R., & Deane, K. (2004). Cancer peer support programs: Do they work? *Patient Education and Counseling*, *55*(1), 3–15. https://doi.org/10.1016/j.pec.2003.10.001

Clougher, D., Ciria-Suarez, L., Medina, J. C., Anastasiadou, D., Racioppi, A., & Ochoa-Arnedo, C. (2023). What works in peer support for breast cancer survivors: A qualitative systematic review and meta-ethnography. *Applied Psychology-Health and Well Being*, *16*(2), 793–815. https://doi.org/10.1111/aphw.12473

D'Egidio, V., Sestili, C., Mancino, M., Sciarra, I., Cocchiara, R., & Backhaus, I., et al. (2017). Counseling interventions delivered in women with breast cancer to improve health-related quality of life: A systematic review. *Quality of Life Research*, *26*, 2573–2592. https://doi.org/10.1007/s11136-017-1613-6

Dunn, J., Steginga, S. K., Rosoman, N., & Millichap, D. (2003). A review of peer support in the context of cancer. *Journal of Psychosocial Oncology*, *21*(2), 55–67. https://doi.org/10.1300/J077v21n02_04

Hatton, R. A., Crane, J., Rogers, S. N., & Patterson, J. (2022). Head and neck cancer peer-to-peer support and quality of life: Systematic scoping review. *British Journal of Nursing*, *31*(5). https://doi.org/10.12968/bjon.2022.31.5.S30

Hoey, L. M., Ieropoli, S. C., White, V. M., & Jefford, M. (2008). Systematic review of peer-support programs for people with cancer. *Patient Education and Counseling*, *70*, 315–337. https://doi.org/10.1016/j.pec.2007.11.016

Hu, J., Wu, Y., Ji, F., Fang, X., & Chen, F. (2020). Peer Support as an ideal solution for racial/ethnic disparities in colorectal cancer screening: Evidence from a systematic review and meta-analysis. *Diseases of the Colon and Rectum*, *63*(6), 850–858. https://doi.org/10.1097/DCR.0000000000001611

Hu, J. M., Wang, X., Guo, S. N., Chen, F. F., Wu, Y. Y., & Ji, F. J., et al. (2019). Peer Support interventions for breast cancer patients: A systematic review. *Breast Cancer Research and Treatment*, *174*, 325–341. https://doi.org/10.1007/s10549-018-5033-2

Ihrig, A., Karschuck, P., Haun, M. W., Thomas, C., & Huber, J. (2020). Online peer-to-peer support for persons affected by prostate cancer: A systematic review. *Patient Education and Counseling*, *103*(10), 2107–2115. https://doi.org/10.1016/j.pec.2020.05.009

Jablotschkin, M., Binkowski, L., Markovits Hoopii, R., & Weis, J. (2022). Benefits and challenges of cancer peer support groups: A systematic review of qualitative studies. *European Journal of Cancer Care*, *31*(6), e13700. https://doi.org/10.1111/ecc.13700

Kiemen, A., Czornik, M., & Weis, J. (2023). How effective is peer-to-peer support in cancer patients and survivors? A systematic review. *Journal of Cancer Research and Clinical Oncology*, *149*, 9461–9485. https://doi.org/10.1007/s00432-023-04753-8

Kowitt, S. D., Ellis, K. R., Carlisle, V., Nivedita, L., Bhushan, N. L., & Black, K. Z., et al. (2019).Peer Support opportunities across the cancer care continuum: A systematic scoping review of recent Peer-reviewed literature. *Support Care Cancer*, *27*(1), 97–108. https://doi.org/10.1007/s00520-018-4479-4

Lee, M. K., & Suh, S. R. (2018). Effects of peer-led interventions for patients with cancer: A meta-analysis. *Oncology Nursing Forum*, *45*(2), 217–236. https://doi.org/10.1188/18.ONF.217-236

Macvean, M. L., White, V. M., & Sanson-Fisher, R. (2008). One-to-one volunteer support programs for people with cancer: A review of the literature. *Patient Education and Counselling*, *70*(1), 10–24. https://doi.org/10.1016/j.pec.2007.08.005

Meyer, A., Coroiu, A., & Korner, A. (2015). One-to-one peer support in cancer care: A review of scholarship published between 2007 and 2014. *European Journal of Cancer Care*, *24*(3), 299–312. https://doi.org/10.1111/ecc.12273

Naung, M. T., Panza, A., Viwattanakulvanid, P., & Htun, Y. Y. (2021). Effect of peer support intervention on quality of life among breast cancer patients on chemotherapy: Intervention and control group study. *Journal of Public Health and Development*, *19*(1), 123–140.

Pefbrianti, D., Suprabawati, D., & Yunitasari, E. (2018). Is peer education an effective method on breast cancers' patient? In *Proceedings of the 9th International Nursing Conference (INC 2018)*, 280–286. https://doi.org/10.5220/0008323902800286

Pyle, D., Perry, A., Lamont-Mills, A., Tehan, G., & Chambers, S. K. (2021). A scoping review of the characteristics and benefits of online prostate cancer communities. *Psycho-Oncology*, *30*(5), 659–668. https://doi.org/10.1002/pon.5618

Que, W. Q., Zhao, J. Y., Tang, J., Su, X. Q., Li, J. M., & Gu, C. H., et al. (2023). Peer supporters' experience of supporting cancer patients: A meta-synthesis. *Cancer Nursing*, *7*(5), E336–E347. https://doi.org/10.1097/NCC.0000000000001214

Sadoh, A. E., Osime, C., Nwaneri, D. U., Ogboghodo, B. C., Eregie, C. O., & Oviawe, O. (2021). Improving knowledge about breast cancer and breast self-examination in female Nigerian adolescents using peer education: A pre-post interventional study. *BMC Women's Health*, *21*, 328. https://doi.org/10.1186/s12905-021-01466-3

Shakya, P., Kunieda, M. K., Koyama, M., Rai, S. S., Miyaguchi, M., & Dhakal, S., et al. (2017). Effectiveness of community-based peer support for mothers to improve their breastfeeding practices: A systematic review and meta-analysis. *Figshare*   https://figshare.com/articles/Effectiveness_of_community-based_peer_support_for_mothers_to_improve_their_breastfeeding_practices_A_systematic_review_and_meta-analysis/5010287

Smith-Turchyn, J., Vani, M. F., Murray, R. M., McCowan, M. E., Edward, H., & Nayiga, B. K., et al. (2023). Peer Support physical activity interventions partnering unknown survivors of cancer: A scoping review. *Rehabilitation Oncology*, *41*(4), 166–179. https://doi.org/10.1097/01.REO.0000000000000343

Tan, Y. Y., Qin, M. J., Liao, B., Wang, L. X., Chang, G. T., & Wei, F. X., et al. (2023). Effectiveness of peer support on quality of life and anxiety in breast cancer patients: A systematic review and meta-analysis. *Breast Care, 18,* 49–58. https://doi.org/10.1159/000527849

Vrontaras, N., Koulierakis, G., Ntourou, I., Karakatsoulis, G., Sergentanis, T., & Kyrou, D., et al. (2023). Psychosocial interventions on the posttraumatic growth of adults with cancer: A systematic review and meta-analysis of clinical trials. *Psycho-Oncology, 32*(12), 1798–1826. https://doi.org/10.1002/pon.6241

Walshe, C., & Roberts, D. (2018). Peer Support for people with advanced cancer: A systematically constructed scoping review of quantitative and qualitative evidence. *Current Opinion in Supportive and Palliative Care, 12*(3), 308–322. https://doi.org/10.1097/SPC.0000000000000370

Walshe, C., Roberts, D., Calman, L., Appleton, L., Croft, R., & Skevington, S., et al. (2019). Peer Support to maintain psychological wellbeing in people with advanced cancer: Findings from a feasibility study for a randomised controlled trial. *BMC Palliative Care, 19,* 129. https://doi.org/10.1186/s12904-020-00631-z

Zhang, S. F., Li, J. J., & Hu, X. (2022). Peer Support interventions on quality of life, depression, anxiety, and self-efficacy among patients with cancer: A systematic review and meta-analysis. *Patient Education and Counseling, 105*(11), 3213–3224. https://doi.org/10.1016/j.pec.2022.07.008

Diabetes

5

DEFINITION

Diabetes is a condition that causes a person's blood sugar level to become too high. There are two main types of diabetes:

- Type 1 diabetes – a lifelong condition where the body's immune system attacks and destroys the cells that produce insulin.
- Type 2 diabetes – where the body does not produce enough insulin, or the body's cells do not react to insulin properly.

Type 2 diabetes is far more common than type 1. In the West, over 90% of all adults with diabetes have type 2.

The amount of sugar in the blood is controlled by a hormone called insulin, which is produced by the pancreas (a gland behind the stomach). When food is digested and enters the bloodstream, insulin moves glucose out of the blood and into cells, where it is broken down to produce energy. However, if you have diabetes, your body is unable to break down glucose into energy. This is because there's either not enough insulin to move the glucose, or the insulin produced does not work properly.

If you have diabetes, your eyes are at risk from diabetic retinopathy, a condition that can lead to sight loss if it's not treated. Diabetes can damage the nerves in your feet and cause a loss of feeling. It can also reduce the blood supply to your feet. This means you may not notice if your foot is sore or injured, and foot injuries do not heal as well. This can lead to ulcers and infections, and sometimes amputations can be needed in serious cases.

Diabetes is more common in people of African or Asian heritage. Peer education/counseling/support for patients with diabetes has been very extensively researched.

DOI: 10.1201/9781003438366-5

REVIEWS OF EVIDENCE

Twenty-seven reviews of research meeting the inclusion criteria were identified. Most of these focused on type 2 diabetes. Three reviews investigated developing countries (Otanga et al., 2022; Pienaar & Reid, 2020; Werfalli et al., 2020). Two reviews investigated digital technology as a means of peer support (Litchman et al., 2020; Titoria et al., 2023).

Loveman et al. (2008) searched databases from 2002 to 2006, including 13 studies. Some trials reported significant improvements on measures of diabetic control but others did not. Some effects were shown on measures of diabetic control in studies that focused on diet or exercise alone. Effects appeared relatively long-lasting. Another review focused on Latinos but only searched one database, including 22 articles (Pérez-Escamilla et al., 2008). Outcome measures included Type 2 diabetes behavioral and metabolic outcomes, nutrition knowledge, attitudes, and behaviors. Peer education had a positive influence on diabetes self-management outcomes, as well as general nutrition knowledge and dietary intake behaviors. Research is needed to identify optimal peer educator characteristics, the type of training that they should receive, the client loads and dosage (i.e., frequency and amount of contact needed between peer educator and client), and the best educational approaches and delivery settings.

Brownson and Heisler (2009) focused on the roles of peers. Peers worked under a variety of titles, which did not define their duties. Providing education and follow-up support were the two most common roles. Mostly, these roles were carried out during face-to-face contact, frequently in community sites. Remaining questions related to cost-effectiveness, sustainability, integration of peers into health and social service delivery systems, and recruitment, training, and support of peers. Five databases were searched by Dale et al. (2012) for 1966–2011. Twenty-five studies, including 14 randomized controlled trials (RCTs), met the inclusion criteria. Peer support showed statistically significant improvements in at least some studies in glycemic control, blood pressure, cholesterol, BMI, weight, physical activity, self-efficacy, depression, and perceived social support.

Kirk et al. (2013) searched three databases from 2006 to mid-2013 for studies conducted in the USA and Europe. The overall trend was that social support could have a positive influence on the ability of the patient to initiate and sustain diabetes management. This appeared true even when the patient had low psychosocial skills and a small social support network.

A meta-analysis conducted by Qi et al. (2015) focused on improving glycemic control. Thirteen RCTs met the inclusion criteria. Peer support resulted in a significant reduction in average blood glucose (sugar) levels HbA1c (Effect Size = 0.57). Programs with moderate or high frequency of contact showed a significant reduction in HbA1c levels, whereas programs with low frequency of contact showed no significant reduction). Those with less glycemic control at baseline were more likely to show effects.

Zhang et al. (2016) noted each 1% reduction in the mean glycemic measure (HbA1c) was associated with reduction in risk of 21% for diabetes, 21% for deaths related to diabetes, 14% for myocardial infarction and 37% for microvascular complications. Seven types of peer support were identified: Have a chat, Support groups, Internet and email peer support, Peer-led groups or events, Individual peer coaches, Telephone-based peer support, Community workers and Service provider-led groups. Three databases were searched and 20 articles were identified up to 2014. Peer support had a significantly positive effect on glycemic control with a pooled effect of 0.16%, $p < 0.001$). Peer support provided by patients themselves or non-professionals had a better effect. The duration of peer support with the best cost-effectiveness was > 3 and ≤ 6 months. Four databases from 1960 to 2015 were searched by Patil et al. (2016), and 17 studies were included. The focus was peer support delivered by people affected by diabetes (those with the disease or a caregiver). There was an improvement in pooled HbA1c level (effect size 0.12, $p = .01$). Peer support showed an HbA1c improvement of 0.48% in the subset of studies with Hispanic participants and 0.53% in the subset of studies with minority participants.

Fisher et al. (2017) searched only one database, including 24 + 30 studies, of which 83% reported significant impacts of peer support, 62% reported between-group differences and 22% reported within-group changes. A median of 65% of the 24 studies reported significant effects of peer support. Of the 30 studies, 26 (87%) reported significant impacts of peer support. Of the 19 reporting HbA1c data, the average reduction was 0.76 points. RCTs between 2006–2016 were reviewed by Gatlin et al. (2017), who included seven studies. There were two types of peer education: face-to-face or a combination of face-to-face and telephone/texting. Two of the six studies showed statistically significant improvement in HbA1c between intervention and control groups. An increase in diabetes knowledge was also statistically significant in two of five studies.

Patil et al. (2018) focused on how peer support by persons affected with diabetes could improve the supporter's diabetes self-management skills. Three databases were searched and 16 articles met inclusion criteria. Outcomes included Body Mass Index (BMI), smoking, diet, physical activity, cholesterol level, glucose control, and blood pressure (BP). There was a positive effect of peer support on systolic BP but a non-significant effect of peer support on diastolic blood pressure, cholesterol, BMI, diet, and physical activity. Six databases were searched by Afshar et al. (2020) and 23 trials were included. Face-to-face was the most common form of contact, although rates of contact were highest for telephone. Potential peer leaders were identified through recommendations from health professionals and were mostly female, university educated, and had a long history of diabetes (≥ 10 years). PL training varied significantly; the two most frequent topics were communication skills and diabetes knowledge. Several studies used methods to evaluate implementation fidelity, but few assessed adherence and competence through audio- and video-taping or direct observations.

Krishnamoorthy et al. (2019) conducted searches in four databases up to 2018 and 29 trials were included. There was a positive effect of peer-led intervention on systolic BP with a pooled effect size of 0.28, but there was significant publication bias. Focusing on peer support, Warshaw et al. (2019) reviewed evidence demonstrating the value of peer support to improve clinical and behavioral outcomes. However, this was a narrative review with little detail of the sources of the papers. A systematic review and meta-analysis of RCTs of diabetes distress was conducted by Kong et al. (2020), who searched six databases up to June 2018, including 13 studies. Peer support intervention did not significantly reduce diabetes distress. This is the only review to fail to find significant results, but it did only focus on diabetic distress. Azmiardi et al. (2021) searched seven databases from 2005 to 2020, including 12 studies. Peer support effectively reduced glycated hemoglobin HbA1c levels (effect size 0.41, p < 0.001). Programs with a sample size < 100, duration of intervention ≤ 6 months, baseline HbA1c < 8.5%, delivery by group and high frequency of contact all had statistically significant effects.

Tang et al. (2011) focused exclusively on interventions involving volunteer peer supporters, searching three databases and including 12 studies with face-to-face and/or telephone contact. Half of the studies gave no payment to peer supporters. Physiological indicators were poor; a minority were effective, but there was much heterogeneity in intervention characteristics (e.g., intervention duration and delivery; peer support selection, recruitment and support structure; roles and responsibilities of peer supporters). A large percentage of studies (33%) compared peers to professionals rather than peers to controls. Nonetheless, peer-led interventions performed as well as professional-led interventions. Eight databases were searched by Liang et al. (2021) to 2019 and 17 studies were included in a meta-analysis. Peer support significantly improved self-efficacy (effect size = 0.41, p = 0.0001) and self-management (effect size = 1.21, p = 0.0002), but had no significant effect on distress (p = 0.34).

Lu et al. (2022) focused on high-income nations, searching four databases between 2007 and 2021 and including 76 records. Face-to-face self-management programs and telephone-based peer support seemed the most promising modalities. Face-to-face self-management programs were the most preferred by ethnic minority groups. Healthcare professionals had mixed views about peer support interventions. Nine databases were searched by Verma et al. (2022), who included 13 RCTs published between 2008 and 2021. There were statistically significant changes in hemoglobin HbA1c. However, there were no significant changes in low-density lipoprotein, BMI, systolic BP or health-related quality of life. However, there were improvements in self-efficacy, diabetes distress and patient activation.

Self-determination theory was used by Helgeson et al. (2023) to understand the conditions under which peer support was helpful or unhelpful. Previous work focused on informational support from peers, which could threaten self-determination needs for autonomy, competence, and relatedness, especially in youth. Chen et al. (2024) focused on the effect of peer support on quality of life, self-management, self-efficacy, glycated hemoglobin (HbA1c) and depression. A systematic review of ten databases from 1974 to mid-2023 was undertaken and 12 studies included. Peer support significantly improved quality of life, self-management, self-efficacy, and HbA1c control, but had no significant effect on depression.

Developing Countries

Three reviews investigated developing countries (Otanga et al., 2022; Pienaar & Reid, 2020; Werfalli et al, 2020).

Pienaar and Reid (2020) researched face-to-face peer support models for adults in low and middle-income countries, searching 15 databases, including Africa-Wide Information, for 2000 to 2017, extracting data from 12 papers. Diabetic patients and community health workers were two common support models. The recruitment and selection of diabetic patients as peer supporters focused on patients with good glycemic control and/or leadership skills, recommended by healthcare professionals. Generally, outcomes were positive. The training of peer supporters was important, with respect to who provided training and the duration and content covered. The supervision of peer supporters was generally poorly described.

Globally, an estimated 380 million people live with diabetes, and 80% of these are in low-income and middle-income countries: the Middle East, Western Pacific, Sub-Saharan Africa, and South-East Asia (Werfalli et al., 2020). Their review focused on community-based peer-led diabetes self-management programs and examined the implementation strategies and outcomes. Eight databases were searched from 2000 to 2019. Eleven studies were included with at least three months of follow-up. Peer support was inconsistently associated with improvements in clinical, behavioral, and psychological outcomes. Many of the studies were of low quality, and most had a substantial risk of bias.

Otanga et al. (2022) researched peer support in Kenya and Uganda. Their scoping review searched three databases between 2000 and 2021, including 13 peer-reviewed articles. Peer support could incorporate group medical visits, diabetes self-management education, telephone support, and Medication Adherence Clubs. Most interventions were effective and led to improvements in HbA1c and BP, eating behaviors and physical activity, and social support.

Digital Technology

Two reviews investigated digital technology as a means of peer support (Litchman et al., 2020; Titoria et al., 2023).

Litchman et al. (2020) conducted a systematic review of reviews from 1978 through 2018, finding 167 reviews, of which nine were included in the study. Findings suggested digital peer support could have a positive impact on clinical outcomes (HbA1C, BP, cholesterol, weight), behavioral outcomes (diabetes knowledge, being active, healthy eating, medication management, self-management, self-efficacy, empowerment), and psychosocial outcomes (social support, health and diabetes distress, depression, quality of life). Technology-mediated peer support for *pediatric* type 1 diabetes was researched by Titoria et al. (2023). Three databases were searched from 2007 to mid-2022, and 12 studies were included, with a duration range of 3 weeks to 24 months. Most were RCTs ($n = 8$). Four technology-based interventions were identified: phone-based text messages, video, web portals, and social media, or a hybrid peer support model. Mixed findings were observed in reduced HbA1c levels ($n = 7$). No significant improvement was observed in psychosocial outcomes (quality of life, stress and coping, social support).

SINGLE STUDIES

Number of Single Studies

One hundred and twenty-six single studies meeting the inclusion criteria were identified, 89 (70%) in developed countries and 37 in developing countries. Given the number of reviews was so large, only four single studies will feature below.

Exemplar Single Studies Developed Context

In China, Liu et al. (2015) aimed to assess the effect of peer education in type 2 diabetes patients with emotional disorders on the physiological meta-bolic index and on psychological status. Psychological scales were used to screen patients with type 2 diabetes and emotional disorders. Participants were divided into peer education and control groups. Both groups received the usual diabetes education from professionals. Peer leaders were recruited to provide support to the peer education group for six months. A total of 127 patients participated. There were 20 peer leaders as volunteers for peer education. The metabolic index, diabetes knowledge, self-management, dia-betes-related distress, emotional status, and quality of life were compared at the end of the study. All participants completed the study and filled the scales. Improvements in the peer education group were significant compared with the usual education control group with respect to anxiety, depression, diabetes knowledge, distress, self-management, and quality of life. However, there was no significant difference in the metabolic index.

Khodneva et al. (2016) examined intervention effects for those with and without depressive symptoms in a peer support trial in the USA. The one-year ENCOURAGE trial included 424 persons with diabetes living in rural Alabama. Intervention participants worked with community volunteers who encouraged participants to engage in daily self-management; control participants received usual clinical care. Outcomes included HbA1c, BMI, and Quality of Life (QoL). Depressive symptoms were assessed with the Patient Health Questionnaire (PHQ). The authors examined control-intervention differences in changes in HbA1c, BMI, and QoL for those with PHQ ≥ 5 and PHQ < 5. Of the 424 par-ticipants enrolled at baseline, 355 completed follow-up and had data that could be included in the study. On average, they were aged 60.2 years, 87% African American, 75% female, and 39% insulin-treated. In the short run, depressive symptoms improved for all, but after 15 months of follow-up intervention, par-ticipants experienced a greater reduction in PHQ score than control participants ($p = 0.01$). Those with PHQ ≥ 5 had unchanged HbA1c, lost weight ($p = 0.03$), and improved QoL ($p = 0.04$). Those with PHQ < 5 also had unchanged HbA1c and lost weight, but did not improve QoL ($p = 0.06$). Peer support improved depres-sive symptoms for all, but resulted in greater weight loss and gains in QoL for those with baseline depressive symptoms compared to those without.

Exemplar Single Studies Developing Context

In Cameroon, Central Africa, Assah et al. (2015) aimed to examine the effec-tiveness of a community-based multilevel peer support intervention in addition to usual diabetes care on improving glycemic levels, BP, and lipids in patients with Type 2 diabetes in Yaoundé. A total of 96 subjects with poorly controlled Type 2 diabetes (intervention group) and 96 age- and sex-matched controls were recruited and followed up over six months. The intervention subjects underwent a peer support intervention through peer-led group meetings, personal encounters, and telephone calls. Both intervention subjects and controls continued their usual clinical care. HbA1c, BP, blood lipids, and self-care behaviors were measured at the outset and six months. There was a significant reduction over six months in HbA1c in the intervention group compared to controls, $p < 0.001$. Peer support also led to significant reductions in fasting blood sugar ($p < 0.001$), cholesterol ($p < 0.001$), high-density cholesterol ($p < 0.001$), BMI ($p < 0.001$), and diastolic BP ($p < 0.001$). Also, diabetes self-care behaviors in the intervention group improved significantly. Thus, community-based peer support, in addition to usual care, significantly improved metabolic control in patients with uncontrolled Type 2 diabetes in Yaoundé.

Khiyali et al. (2021) reported a study carried out in Iran, aiming to investigate the effect of peer group intervention on self-care behaviors and glycemic index in the elderly with type II diabetes mellitus. A quasi-experimental study was conducted on 100 elderly patients with type II diabetes (50 patients in the intervention group and 50 in the control group). In addition to the usual care of the diabetes clinic, the patients in the intervention group received training from their peers for eight weeks during eight 45-minute training sessions. A valid self-report questionnaire was used, including demographic variables, awareness, and diabetes self-care behaviors. In addition, fasting blood sugar and hemoglobin HbA1c were tested in both groups before and two months after the intervention. The results showed that the two groups of intervention and control were initially identical. In the intervention group, after two months of peer education intervention, there was a significant difference in awareness and self-care behaviors in diet, physical activity, blood sugar testing, foot care, and medication (all $p < 0.001$). In the intervention group, the mean fasting blood sugar and quarterly HbA1c index decreased significantly ($p < 0.05$).

SPECIFIC PROGRAM

The specific program reported here is actually the protocol for a randomized controlled trial, but the final results are not yet available (Seuring, et al., 2019). However, it is one of the few reports from a developing country which gives adequate details of implementation.

In Indonesia, diabetes has become one of the main contributors to the burden of disease, surpassing many communicable diseases, especially among adults. However, diabetes treatment at the main public primary-care facilities, puskesmas, remains poor, which is partly due to the limited knowledge of healthcare professionals about diabetes. Consequently, recent studies on diabetes in Indonesia indicate poor levels of control, with around 70% of patients having glycated hemoglobin (HbA1c) levels above 7%. Each puskesmas normally serves one subdistrict, which has a population of 30,000 to 50,000. Peer education groups were randomly established in 50% of puskesmas after they joined the study.

Effectiveness

This study will investigate the effectiveness of peer education over a relatively long time of 18 months. It further aims not only to look at HbA1c, but also at changes in lipid levels as well as BP and waist circumference. The personal characteristics of study participants will also be assessed. The primary outcome is the change in HbA1c levels from baseline to the final assessment. HbA1c will be collected at baseline, midline, and the final assessment. Secondary outcomes are changes in lipids (total cholesterol, high-density lipoprotein, and triglycerides), and at the final assessment: BP, waist circumference, diabetes knowledge, medication adherence (five-item Medication Adherence Scale, MARS-5), diabetes distress (Diabetes Distress Scale 2), health behaviors, such as smoking status and number of cigarettes per day, and physical activity levels (WHO global physical activity questionnaire), and dietary diversity (dietary diversity questionnaire published by the Food and Agriculture Organization of the U.N.). Regarding the behavioral characteristics of the participants, we measure risk and time preferences as well as trust in other people. We also use the Collective Self-Esteem Scale (which measures the ability of participants to function in and identify with social groups) and the 13-item Self-Control Scale. Finally, to assess the cost-effectiveness of the intervention, changes in healthcare costs and changes in quality-adjusted life years (based on EQ-5D-3 L questionnaire) will be used.

Implementation

The intervention was designed in cooperation with the local expert team as well as experts experienced with the implementation of peer education in a low-income context in Mali. Furthermore, qualitative interviews and focus group discussions with nurses working with diabetes patients at puskesmas informed the intervention design, in particular regarding practicable ways to train peer educators and to provide them with the means to transfer their knowledge successfully to their peer groups.

The peer educators will need to fulfill the following requirements: can commit to attending 20 hours of training, are willing to organize activities with other patients every month, have basic diabetes self-management knowledge and supportive non-judgmental communication skills, be willing to lead and be literate. Peer educators will receive training before and after the start of the intervention. A two-day intensive training session by local physicians on diabetes and nutrition was carried out before the start of the peer education sessions. It provided general information about diabetes as a disease, its risks, and the ways to treat it. This will be followed up by monthly half-day training sessions for the peer educators until the end of the study. These training sessions will be led by two specially trained nurses, who will be educated by a member of the research team on the specific topic to be discussed. The topics and structure of the peer educator training sessions will be guided by the peer leader manual published by the International Diabetes Federation.

At baseline, the patients recruited were interviewed. They were invited to the puskesmas, during which their HbA1c and lipid levels were tested. Participants were informed of their test results. In choosing potential peer educators, all participants were asked during the interviews if they would be interested in serving as a peer educator. Further, health facility staff were asked to suggest patients for this role. Depending on the number of patients recruited per puskesmas and the number of potential peer educators, one or two peer educators will be selected per puskesmas, to limit the group size to 13 participants. Peer education sessions are planned to be held once a month for 18 months. They will be conducted by the peer educator only, without the presence of a trained nurse or a member of the research staff. No implementation integrity checks were proposed; but feedback from the peer educators. Patients with diabetes were recruited into the peer education program. The researchers determined potential peer educators based on three criteria: (1) their willingness to take on this role, (2) a recommendation from the health facility staff, and (3) how well they were already controlling their diabetes based on the HbA1c level from the baseline data.

REFERENCES

Afshar, R., Tang, T. S., Askari, A. S., Sidhu, R., Brown, H., & Sherifali, D. (2020). Peer Support interventions in type 2 diabetes: Review of components and process outcomes. *Journal of Diabetes*, *12*(4), 315–338. https://doi.org/10.1111/1753-0407.12999

Assah, F. K., Atanga, E. N., Enoru, S., Sobngwi, E., & Mbanya, J. C. (2015). Community-based peer support significantly improves metabolic control in people with type 2 diabetes in Yaoundé, Cameroon. *Diabetic Medicine: A Journal of the British Diabetic Association, 32*(7), 886–889. https://doi.org/10.1111/dme.12720

Azmiardi, A., Murti, B., Febrinasari, R. P., & Tamtomo, D. G. (2021). The effect of peer support in diabetes self-management education on glycemic control in patients with type 2 diabetes: A systematic review and meta-analysis. *Epidemiology and Health, 43*, e2021090. https://doi.org/10.4178/epih.e2021090

Brownson, C. A., & Heisler, M. (2009). The role of peer support in diabetes care and self-management. *Patient, 2*(1), 5–17. https://doi.org/10.2165/01312067-200902010-00002

Chen, C., Zhou, Y., Xu, J. Y., Song, H. Y., Yin, X. W., & Gu, Z. J. (2024). Effect of peer support interventions in patients with type 2 diabetes: A systematic review. *Patient Education and Counseling, 122*, 108172. https://doi.org/10.1016/j.pec.2024.108172

Dale, J. R., Williams, S. M., & Bowyer, V. (2012). What is the effect of peer support on diabetes outcomes in adults? A systematic review. *Diabetic Medicine, 29*, 1361–1377. https://doi.org/10.1111/j.1464-5491.2012.03749.x

Fisher, E. B., Boothroyd, R. I., Elstad, E. A., Hays, L., Henes, A., Maslow, G. R., & Velicer, C. (2017). Peer Support of complex health behaviors in prevention and disease management with special reference to diabetes: Systematic reviews. *Clinical Diabetes and Endocrinology, 25*(3), 4. https://doi.org/10.1186/s40842-017-0042-3

Gatlin, T. K., Serafica, R., & Johnson, M. (2017). Systematic review of peer education intervention programmes among individuals with type 2 diabetes. *Journal of Clinical Nursing, 26*, 4212–4222. https://doi.org/10.1111/jocn.13991

Helgeson, V. S., Berg, C. A., & Raymaekers, K. (2023). Topical review: Youth with type 1 diabetes: What is the role of Peer support? *Journal of Pediatric Psychology, 48*(2), 176–180. https://doi.org/10.1093/jpepsy/jsac083

Khiyali, Z., Ghasemi, A., Toghroli, R., Ziapour, A., Shahabi, N., & Dehghan, A., et al. (2021). The effect of peer group on self-care behaviors and glycemic index in elders with type II diabetes. *Journal of Education and Health Promotion, 10*, 197. https://doi.org/10.4103/jehp.jehp_990_20

Khodneva, Y., Safford, M. M., Richman, J., Gamboa, C., Andreae, S., & Cherrington, A. (2016). Volunteer peer support, diabetes, and depressive symptoms: Results from the ENCOURAGE trial. *Journal of Clinical & Translational Endocrinology, 4*, 38–44. https://doi.org//10.1016/j.jcte.2016.04.002

Kirk, J. K., Ebert, C. N., Gamble, G. P., & Ebert, E. C. (2013). Social support strategies in adult patients with diabetes: A review of strategies in the USA and Europe. *Expert Review of Endocrinology & Metabolism, 8*(4), 379–389. https://doi.org/10.1586/17446651.2013.811895

Kong, L. N., Hu, P., Zhao, Q. H., Yao, H. Y., & Chen, S. Z. (2020). Effect of peer support intervention on diabetes distress in people with type 2 diabetes: A systematic review and meta-analysis. *International Journal of Nursing Practice, 26*(5), e12830. https://doi.org/10.1111/ijn.12830

Krishnamoorthy, Y., Sakthivel, M., Sarveswaran, G., & Eliyas, S. K. (2019). Effectiveness of peer led intervention in improvement of clinical outcomes among diabetes mellitus and hypertension patients: A systematic review and meta-analysis. *Primary Care Diabetes*, *13*(2), 158–169. https://doi.org/10.1016/j.pcd.2018.11.007

Liang, D. D., Jia, R. Y., Zhou, X., Lu, G. L., Wu, Z., Yu, J. F., Wang, Z. H., Huang, H. T., Guo, J. Y., & Chen, C. R. (2021). The effectiveness of peer support on self-efficacy and self-management in people with type 2 diabetes: A meta-analysis. *Patient Education and Counseling*, *104*(4), 760–769. https://doi.org/10.1016/j.pec.2020.11.011

Litchman, M. L., Oser, T. K., Hodgson, L., Heyman, M., Walker, H. R., Deroze, P., Rinker, J., & Warshaw, H. (2020). In-person and technology-mediated Peer support in diabetes care: A systematic review of reviews and gap analysis. *The Diabetes Educator*, *46*(3), 230–241. https://doi.org/10.1177/0145721720913275

Liu, Y., Han, Y., Shi, J., Li, R. X., Li, S. F., Jin, N. N., Gu, Y., & Guo, H. L. (2015). Effect of peer education on self-management and psychological status in type 2 diabetes patients with emotional disorders. *Journal of Diabetes Investigation*, *6*, 479–486. https://doi.org/10.1111/jdi.12311

Loveman, E., Frampton, G. K., & Clegg, A. J. (2008). The clinical effectiveness of diabetes education models for type 2 diabetes: A systematic review. *Health Technology Assessment*, *12*(9), 1–136. https://doi.org/10.3310/hta12090

Lu, S., Leduc, N., & Moullec, G. (2022). Type 2 diabetes peer support interventions as a complement to primary care settings in high-income nations: A scoping review. *Patient Education and Counseling*, *105*(11), 3267–3278. https://doi.org/10.1016/j.pec.2022.08.010

Otanga, H., Semujju, B., Mwaniki, L., & Aungo, J. (2022). Peer Support and social networking interventions in diabetes self-management in Kenya and Uganda: A scoping review. *PLoS One*, *17*(9), e0273722. https://doi.org/10.1371/journal.pone.0273722

Patil, S. J., Ruppar, T., Koopman, R. J., Lindbloom, E. J., Elliott, S. G., Mehr, D. R., & Conn, V. S. (2016). Peer Support interventions for adults with diabetes: A meta-analysis of hemoglobin A_{1c} outcomes. *Annals of Family Medicine*, *14*(6), 540–551. https://doi.org/10.1370/afm.1982

Patil, S. J., Ruppar, T., Koopman, R. J., Lindbloom, E. J., Elliott, S. G., Mehr, D. R., & Conn, V. S. (2018). Effect of peer support interventions on cardiovascular disease risk factors in adults with diabetes: A systematic review and meta-analysis. *BMC Public Health*, *18*, 398. https://doi.org/10.1186/s12889-018-5326-8

Pérez-Escamilla, R., Hromi-Fiedler, A., Vega-López, S., Bermúdez-Millán, A., & Segura-Pérez, S. (2008). Impact of peer nutrition education on dietary behaviors and health outcomes among Latinos: A systematic literature review. *Journal of Nutrition Education and Behavior*, *40*, 208–225. https://doi.org/10.1016/j.jneb.2008.03.011

Pienaar, M., & Reid, M. (2020). Self-management in face-to-face peer support for adults with type 2 diabetes living in low- or middle-income countries: A systematic review. *BMC Public Health*, *20*, 1834. https://doi.org/10.1186/s12889-020-09954-1

Qi, L., Liu, Q., Qi, X., Wu, N., Tang, W., & Xiong, H. (2015). Effectiveness of peer support for improving glycaemic control in patients with type 2 diabetes: A meta-analysis of randomized controlled trials. *BMC Public Health*, *15*, 471. https://doi.org/10.1186/s12889-015-1798-y

Seuring, T., Marthoenis, S. R., Rogge, L., Rau, H., Besançon, S., Zufry, H., Sofyan, H., & Vollmer, S. (2019). Using peer education to improve diabetes management and outcomes in a low-income setting: A randomized controlled trial. *Trials*, *20*, 548. https://doi.org/10.1186/s13063-019-3656-1

Tang, T. S., Ayala, G. X., Cherrington, A., & Rana, G. (2011). A review of volunteer-based peer support interventions in diabetes. *Diabetes Spectrum*, *24*(2). 85–98. https://doi.org/10.2337/diaspect.24.2.85

Titoria, R., Fung, A., Tang, T. S., & Amed, S. (2023). Systematic review of technology-mediated peer support interventions in paediatric type 1 diabetes care. *Diabetic Medicine: A Journal of the British Diabetic Association*, *40*(10), e15172. https://doi.org/10.1111/dme.15172

Verma, I., Gopaldasani, V., Jain, V., Chauhan, S., Chawla, R., Verma, P. K., & Hosseinzadeh, H. (2022). The impact of peer coach-led type 2 diabetes mellitus interventions on glycaemic control and self-management outcomes: A systematic review and meta-analysis. *Primary Care Diabetes*, *16*(6), 719–735. https://doi.org/10.1016/j.pcd.2022.10.007

Warshaw, H., Hodgson, L., Heyman, M., Oser, T. K., Walker, H. R., Deroze, P., Rinker, J., & Litchman, M. L. (2019). The role and value of ongoing and peer support in diabetes care and education. *The Diabetes Educator*, *45*(6), 569–579. https://doi.org/10.1177/0145721719882007

Werfalli, M., Raubenheimer, P. J., Engel, M., Musekiwa, A., Bobrow, K., Peer, N., Hoegfeldt, C., Kalula, S., Kengne, A. P., & Levitt, N. S. (2020). The effectiveness of peer and community health worker-led self-management support programs for improving diabetes health-related outcomes in adults in low- and middle-income countries: A systematic review. *Systematic Reviews*, *9*, 133. https://doi.org/10.1186/s13643-020-01377-8

Zhang, X, X., Yang, S. S., Sun, K., Fisher, E. B., & Sun, X. Y. (2016). How to achieve better effect of peer support among adults with type 2 diabetes: A meta-analysis of randomized clinical trials. *Patient Education and Counseling*, *99*(2), 186–197. https://doi.org/10.1016/j.pec.2015.09.006

Neurological, Heart and Other Conditions

6

DEFINITION

This chapter mainly explores peer interventions in six areas: chronic health conditions, spinal cord injury, heart conditions, neurological conditions, stroke, and asthma, listed in the order of number of reviews of papers concerning them.

Chronic Health Conditions

Chronic diseases are defined broadly as conditions that cannot currently be cured and last one year or more, requiring ongoing medical attention and/or limiting activities of daily living. They include diseases mentioned separately (below and elsewhere) such as arthritis, chronic fatigue, and high blood pressure, all characterized by their longevity.

Spinal Cord Injury

After spinal cord injury, damaged nerves are unable to generate or carry signals up or down beyond the point of injury, and the injured person loses sensory information and muscle control. This lack of communication affects everyday living in many ways, such as touch, grip, temperature, breathing, bladder control, swallowing, talking, blood pressure, and sexual function. In the majority of cases, the damage results from physical trauma. The most commonly affected group are young adult males. This area really belongs to neurological disorders (below).

DOI: 10.1201/9781003438366-6

Heart Conditions

Heart disease (or cardiovascular disease) includes blood vessel disease (such as coronary artery disease), irregular heartbeats (arrhythmias), heart problems present from birth (congenital heart defects), disease of the heart muscle (cardiomyopathy), and heart valve disease. Angina, heart attack (myocardial infarction), and heart failure can result.

Neurological Conditions

Neurological disorders affect the brain as well as the nerves found throughout the human body. Some of the most common are epilepsy, Alzheimer's disease and other dementias, migraine and other headaches, multiple sclerosis, Parkinson's disease, neurological infections, brain tumors, and traumatic head injuries.

Stroke

A stroke is a loss of blood flow to part of the brain, which damages brain tissue. Strokes are caused by blood clots and bleeding in the brain. Common symptoms include face drooping on one side, not being able to lift arms, and slurred speech. A transient ischemic attack (also called a TIA or "mini-stroke") is similar, but the blood flow to the brain is only temporarily disrupted. This area relates to both cardiovascular disease and neurological disorders.

Asthma

Asthma is a condition in which airways narrow and swell and may produce extra mucus. This can make breathing difficult and trigger coughing, a whistling sound (wheezing) when breathing out, and shortness of breath.

REVIEWS OF EVIDENCE

There were 34 reviews in total. Again, the areas are listed in order of number of reviews of papers concerning them. There were also single reviews of rheumatic diseases and kidney diseases.

Chronic Health Conditions

There were 11 reviews in this area. Three reviews focused on adolescents and school-related issues. Canter and Roberts (2012) reviewed the effects of school re-entry interventions, examining illness- or injury-specific knowledge among teachers and healthy peers, attitudinal change toward an ill or injured child, and the ill or injured child's global self-worth. Larger effect sizes (ES) were found for increases in knowledge than for positive attitudinal changes (mean ES for knowledge: 0.86, mean ES for positive attitudinal change: 0.68). There was a small effect on self-worth (mean ES = 0.24). Community-based mentoring and peer-led programs intending to increase the quality of life for adolescents with chronic illnesses were examined by Merianos et al. (2016). Six articles were included in the narrative analysis. The interventions yielded promising results. Runions et al. (2020) examined research on the experiences of schools for children with chronic health conditions in a scoping review. Two databases were searched and 38 articles were selected. Absenteeism due to illness or healthcare, self-perceived differences from peers, stigmatization and discrimination, bullying and victimization, and positive aspects of peer support at school were reviewed. School-based social risk processes are likely to contribute to psychological problems, and these risks could not be disentangled from mesosystemic, exosystemic, and macrosystemic influences.

One review focused on the elderly (Moore et al., 2021). Three databases were searched in 2018 for randomized controlled trials (RCTs). In 28 included studies, volunteers provided a range of roles (e.g., counsellors, educators, and coaches) with seniors with a variety of chronic conditions (e.g., dementia, diabetes) and health states (e.g., frail, palliative). Volunteers could improve both physical function and physical activity levels.

Four reviews addressed peer interventions with chronic health conditions in general. McBrien et al. (2018) searched six databases in 2017, selecting 67 studies. Of these, 44 were in cancer, eight in diabetes, seven in HIV/AIDS, four in cardiovascular disease, two in chronic kidney disease, one in dementia, and one in patients with multiple conditions. Forty-five of 67 studies reported a statistically significant improvement in the primary outcome. Outlining successful components of any intervention was required. Online support groups (OSGs) for musculoskeletal conditions were studied by Maclachlan et al. (2020). Six databases were searched in 2018, and 21 studies were selected. Of these, 13 studies included OSGs hosted on public platforms, 11 studies examined OSGs conducted in English, and six studies used moderators or peer leaders to facilitate engagement. The majority of OSG members were females who were not full-time employees. Studies identified empowerment, social support, self-management behavior, and health literacy as primary constructs to measure OSG efficacy. Neutral or marginal improvement was reported in these. A greater level of engagement had an important influence on efficacy.

Price et al. (2022) aimed to map the volume, diversity, and nature of high-quality evidence on the effectiveness and cost-effectiveness of peer support, searching 11 databases and selecting 91 studies, including 32 systematic reviews, 52 RCTs, and seven economic evaluations. Studies had been conducted in high-income countries since 2015. The majority of studies measured health-related indicators as outcomes; few studies assessed cost-effectiveness. There was substantial evidence from RCTs for several types of peer intervention: education, coaching, and mentoring; psychological, emotional and well-being support; self-care and self-management; and social and community. A systematic review of reviews was conducted by Thompson et al. (2022), who selected 31 publications. Components of peer intervention were: social support, psychological support, practical support, empowerment, condition monitoring and treatment adherence, informational support, behavioral change, encouragement and motivation, and physical training. Quality of life and self-efficacy were the most measured outcome domains. Most reviews reported positive but non-significant effects.

Two papers specifically looked at peer support delivered through technology. Hossain et al. (2021) searched five databases looking for peer support delivered via the web, selecting 41 articles. There were few RCTs and few studies with older participants. Four of the six RCTs reported positive and significant results, including decreased emotional distress, better health service navigation, and improved self-efficacy. Berkanish et al. (2022) focused on adolescents, selecting 32 papers. The most common technologies were websites with discussion forums ($n = 18$), chat messaging ($n = 9$), and video conferencing ($n = 7$). Results supported the feasibility and acceptability of these interventions, and suggested positive effects on social support, but were mixed on isolation, quality of life, and disease self-management.

Implementation in low- and middle-income countries was reviewed by Graham et al. (2016), searching two databases and identifying 71 papers addressing eight chronic conditions; two chronic communicable diseases (HIV and TB) accounted for the majority of papers ($n = 37$, 52%). Nine (13%) papers reported the use of a package of care provision strategies (mostly related to HIV and/or TB in sub-Saharan Africa). Most papers addressed a narrow aspect of clinical care provision, such as patient education ($n = 23$). Low-income countries were underrepresented ($n = 24$, 34%), almost exclusively involving HIV interventions in sub-Saharan Africa ($n = 21$).

Spinal Cord Injury

There were eight reviews in this area – a lot considering the relative infrequency of the condition. Wobma et al. (2016) searched five databases in 2015 and selected two RCTs, which suggested a positive influence of peer support for traumatic brain injury survivors in social support, coping, behavioral control, and physical quality of life. A scoping review by Barclay and Hilton (2019) on peer support via videoconferencing searched four databases in 2018 and included 21 studies, of which two were RCTs. There was variation in the description and duration of the interventions. The majority were one-to-one ($n = 15$). Beaudoin et al. (2020) focused on mobility, searching four databases and selecting 13 studies, including RCTs. Six peer-led studies evaluated participation and two evaluated mobility. Some studies reported high effect sizes, but others found no significant differences between intervention and control groups. A scoping review was conducted by Chaffey and Bigby (2018) and selected eight studies. Half of these studies included peer education as one component of a broader program, but all reported positive participant outcomes.

McIntyre et al. (2020) also conducted a scoping review, searching five databases and including 112 studies of 102 self-management programs. The majority of the programs took an individual approach (52.0%) as opposed to a group (27.4%) or mixed approach (17.6%). Components included symptom management ($n = 44$; 43%), information about condition/treatment ($n = 34$; 33%), coping ($n = 33$; 32%), training/rehearsal for psychological strategies ($n = 52$; 51%), and lifestyle advice and support ($n = 52$; 510%), taking action ($n = 62$; 61%), and resource utilization ($n = 57$; 56%). A synthesis of 21 qualitative peer-reviewed studies and 66 community documents was conducted by Rocchi et al. (2022). A total of 87 outcomes of peer mentorship were identified, grouped into six themes: 1) Independence: enhanced self-sufficiency; 2) Personal growth: positive psychological changes; 3) Activities and participation: greater participation in activities and events; 4) Adaptation: adapting to life with a disability; 5) Knowledge: obtaining new information, resources, and opportunities; and 6) Connection: developing and maintaining a social relationship. Participating in peer mentorship could promote improved health and quality of life.

Wasilewski et al. (2023) also conducted a scoping review of 93 articles. Most peer support programs provide one-on-one support from peer mentors using various modalities. Interventions were successful when they involved knowledgeable peer mentors and maintained participant engagement. Prior negative experiences and stigma/privacy concerns deterred trauma survivors from participating. A systematic review by Wedege et al. (2024)

searched seven databases and selected ten studies: five qualitative, four quantitative, and one mixed method. Programs lasted from two to 17 days and all addressed independence, health, or quality of life. Program participation positively impacted cognition, emotions, independence, and social life. The evidence on life satisfaction and community participation was inconclusive.

Heart Conditions

There were four reviews in this area (but a great many individual papers). Parry and Watt-Watson (2010) searched nine databases and selected 27 studies, of which only six met the inclusion criteria. Some positive effects of peer support for individuals with heart disease were found, including higher levels of self-efficacy, improved activity, reduced pain, and fewer emergency room visits. A systematic review was conducted by Palacios et al. (2017) to (1) determine the effectiveness of internet-delivered self-management support, on mood, and self-management-related outcomes, and (2) identify and describe essential components for effectiveness. Three databases were searched and seven studies were selected. All reported significant positive effects, in particular for lifestyle-related outcomes.

Hosseinzadeh et al. (2019) searched five databases up to 2018. Peer education had three components: Self-care, Quality of life, and Self-efficacy, and had a positive effect on all three. It was an effective and cost-effective method without the need for specialized equipment. A systematic review and meta-analysis were conducted by Nakao et al. (2023), searching five databases to 2022 and including three studies, including RCTs. Peer support resulted in a reduction in the readmission rate and an improvement in quality of life (effect size 2.03 but very low certainty of the evidence).

Neurological Conditions

There were four reviews in this area. Morris et al. (2017) searched 14 databases plus gray literature sources in 2016 for one-to-one peer mentoring, selecting six studies, including two RCTs. Significant improvements were shown in behavioral control, mood, coping, and quality of life. No significant improvements in social activity level or social network size were found. The impact of peer support for adults on quality of life was investigated by Levy et al. (2019), who scrutinized four databases for RCTs from 2009 to 2019 and selected six studies. Two found significant improvements in quality of life. Hughes et al. (2020) investigated peer support groups, searching four databases and selecting 13 papers. The experience of a peer support group was largely found to be positive. The benefits of peer support were being connected, interacting with others, and providing and receiving support. A scoping review by Aterman et al. (2023) searched four databases in 2021 and selected 53 articles. Peer interventions varied significantly, including individual and group-based formats delivered in-person, by telephone, or online. Content varied from structured education to tailored approaches. Participant outcomes included improved health, confidence, and self-management skills.

Stroke

There were two reviews in this area. Clark et al. (2020) searched four databases in 2017, selecting 12 studies and eight different self-management interventions. Key features were: increasing knowledge, collaboration and/or communication, accessing resources, goal setting, and problem-solving. Peer support facilitated the sharing of experiences, social comparison, vicarious learning, and increased motivation. Peer support interventions for the physical and psychosocial outcomes of stroke survivors were systematically and meta-analyzed by Wan et al. (2021), who searched 11 databases and selected 11 studies. Peer support interventions could improve daily living activities (p = 0.03), limb function, depression (p = 0.006), and anxiety. Social participation (p = 0.03) and quality of life (p = 0.01) also improved.

Asthma

There were two reviews in this area. Kew et al. (2017) searched a trials register to 2016, selecting five studies including RCTs. All participants were 11–17 years of age. Primary outcomes were quality of life and exacerbations requiring at least oral steroids. The duration was 2½ to 9 months, and settings varied (school, day camp, primary care) as did intervention content. Three studies used the Triple A program. Quality of life showed a small benefit. Effects on asthma control favored the intervention but were not statistically significant. Results from two studies with high levels of baseline smoking showed some promise for self-efficacy to stop smoking. Sixteen databases were searched by Zhong and Melendez-Torres (2017) to 2015 for RCTs, including participants aged 10–19 years old. Four studies were selected. There was a small, non-significant increase in participants' quality of life and a small non-significant decrease in lung function. In one RCT, interventions reduced asthma symptoms and improved self-management.

Single Reviews

There were also single reviews of rheumatic diseases and kidney diseases. Karp et al. (2023) investigated rheumatic diseases. Generally, patients across the spectrum of rheumatic disease perceived peer support as a useful tool. Peer support interventions, while highly variable, were generally associated with positive impacts on health-related quality of life metrics (both perceived and measured), although these differences were not always statistically significant. Important limitations included selection bias among study participants and short follow-up periods. Patients with kidney failure undergoing kidney replacement therapy were investigated by Longley et al. (2023), who searched five databases and selected 12 studies (eight RCTs, one quasi-experimental controlled trial, and three single-arm trials). Three studies highlighted the links between peer support and improved patient engagement with care, while one found peer support did not significantly impact engagement. Three studies showed associations between peer support and improvements in psychological well-being. Four studies underscored the effects of peer support on self-efficacy and one on treatment adherence.

SINGLE STUDIES

Number of Single Studies

There were six single studies on Chronic Health Conditions, 18 on Spinal Cord Injury, 32 on Heart Conditions, four on Stroke, and ten on Asthma. In addition, there were some papers on single studies of other medical conditions (three on kidney disease, and one each on urinary tract infections, atrophic gastritis, and autism), which are detailed in the appendix. Here one paper in each main area will be described, rather than the developing/developed categorization seen in previous chapters. The vast majority of papers came from developed countries and did not target disadvantaged samples.

Chronic Health Conditions

Depping et al. (2021) evaluated the efficacy of a brief peer-delivered intervention for patients with rare diseases, including neurofibromatosis type 1, Marfan syndrome, primary sclerosing cholangitis, and pulmonary arterial hypertension. Eighty-nine patients were randomized, of whom 87 completed the six-month follow-up assessment. The six-week peer intervention consisted of a self-help book and telephone-based peer counseling. Peer counselors received training, structured consultation guidelines, and supervision. Six months after the intervention, the intervention group had significantly higher rates of acceptance of the disease (p = 0.01). Several secondary outcomes, including different coping strategies, social support, and mental quality of life, were also significantly higher after the intervention compared with the control group.

Spinal Cord Injury

Two of the 18 single study papers were from developing countries. The effectiveness of peer interventions on self-efficacy, unplanned hospital readmissions, and quality of life for patients with spinal cord injury (SCI) undergoing inpatient rehabilitation were examined by Jones et al. (2021). Participants were 1,117 inpatients admitted for rehabilitation whose discharge location was home (mostly male). A subsample of 799 patients participated in secondary analyses. The intervention was one-to-one mentoring and participation in peer-led self-management classes. Outcome measures were: unplanned readmissions, general self-efficacy, and depressive symptoms 30-, 90- and 180-days post-discharge, plus satisfaction with life at 180 days. There was a significant decrease in both level and slope of readmissions. Reduction in the number of unplanned hospital days was associated with a number of peer visits but not peer-led education classes attended. Higher self-efficacy was associated with greater exposure to peer mentoring, and a significant relationship between improved self-efficacy and reduced readmission was observed.

Heart Conditions

Twelve of the 32 single papers came from developing countries. Wang and Guo (2019) sought to explore the effect of peer education among discharged patients after mechanical heart valve replacement with 84 patients, divided into intervention and control. The experimental group was given peer education from one month to six months after discharge. Anti-coagulant knowledge, anti-coagulant therapy compliance, and complication rates were compared between the two groups, one, three, and six months after discharge. The anti-coagulant knowledge and anti-coagulant therapy compliance of the experimental group were higher than those of the control group at all time intervals after the intervention (p < 0.01), and the incidence of complications was lower than that of the control group at six months (p < 0.01). At six months, the incidence of complications in the experimental group was lower than that in the control group (p < 0.05).

Stroke

Kronish et al. (2014) aimed to reduce disparities in recurrent stroke among Black and Latino stroke survivors, enrolling 600 stroke or transient ischemic attack survivors from diverse low-income communities. A randomized trial compared a six-week (1 session per week) peer-led community-based stroke prevention self-management group workshop (n = 301) to a waitlist control group (n = 299). The primary outcome was the proportion with a composite of controlled blood pressure, low-density lipoprotein cholesterol, and use of antithrombotic medications at six months. Secondary outcomes included control of individual stroke risk factors. The proportion with controlled blood pressure at six months was greater in the intervention group than in the control group (p = 0.02), and there was also a greater change in systolic blood pressure (p = 0.04). There were no group differences in the control of cholesterol or use of anti-thrombotics.

Asthma

The effect of a peer-led program for asthma education on quality of life and related morbidity in adolescents with asthma was conducted by Shah et al. (2001). Students from six high schools in rural Australia (n = 272) with recent wheeze were recruited from two school years (mean age 12.5 and 15.5 years) – 251 completed the study. The "Triple A" peer education program was used. Outcome measures were quality of life, school absenteeism, asthma attacks and lung function. Mean quality of life scores showed significant improvement in the intervention than the control group. Clinically important improvement in quality of life occurred in 25% of students with asthma in the intervention group compared with 12% in the control group (p = 0.01). The effect of the intervention was greatest in students in year 10 and in females. However, significant improvements occurred in the activities domain (41% vs. 28%) and in the emotions domain (39% vs. 19%) in males in the intervention group. School absenteeism significantly decreased in the intervention group only. Asthma attacks at school increased in the control group only.

SPECIFIC PROGRAM

The specific program was taken from a developed country and focused on heart conditions. However, many of these papers included limited descriptions of the peer education, counseling or support procedures. An exception was that of Willock et al. (2015). African American women suffer disproportionately from heart disease mortality and morbidity.

Effectiveness

Training resulted in appreciable effects on four of five outcome measures. Heart health knowledge increased significantly among experienced peer Community Health Workers (CHWs). They were satisfied with training, and training retention was 100%. They initiated and subsequently delivered 122 person-hours of community heart health education and CHW training in their local communities up to 90 days after training.

Implementation

A Learning Circle approach was used to train CHWs. The curriculum blended web-based, self-directed learning and in-person peer coaching. CHWs learned through (a) peer-to-peer sharing, (b) problem-solving and brainstorming, and (c) leadership and experiential activities. The training used the National Heart, Lung, and Blood Institute *With Every Heartbeat Is Life: A Community Health Worker's Manual for African Americans*. The CHWs were involved in stages of change assessments, behavior change strategies, and active listening. Participatory learning was used, encouraging participants to share their opinions, generate innovative ideas, make informed decisions, evaluate personal experiences, make training enjoyable, and apply principles learned to everyday life.

The peer-to-peer training model was selected over more traditional formal models because it most closely approximated the typical facilitation styles of CHWs. It also promoted the rapid assimilation of large amounts of new information since CHWs were actively engaged and learned through their own experiences, getting relevant skill practice with support and input from their peers and a master facilitator. Participatory peer-led learning offered a reciprocal teaching–learning relationship where the facilitation process enhanced both the individual doing the teaching and the one being taught.

Few previous reports identify peer-to-peer participatory training approaches as the primary CHW training method.

Recruitment included engaging with community-based and faith-based organizations that had existing relationships with CHWs, recruitment of CHWs, CHW résumé review and interview, and CHW selection and invitation to training. Recruitment was through the Georgia Community Health Workers Network e-mail list and through the newsletter of an academic medical center that regularly uses CHWs. Recruitment was also conducted through presentations, referrals from Georgia Department of Public Health District Officers, and other organizations. Forty-four CHWs responded to recruitment, and 37 eligible CHWs completed the application process.

Twenty-five CHWs were selected to receive the training. The selection process included a review of CHWs' experience, their performance in a phone interview, and a letter of support. Each training cycle required a 28-hour time commitment over 2 weeks and provided CHWs with a stipend. The Learning Circle supported participation from all CHWs while providing participants with heart health content, tools to assimilate and subsequently communicate heart health information, and the confidence to be an engaged peer learner. The peer-led learner experience was modeled so that CHWs learned through (a) peer sharing and listening, (b) problem-solving and problem-posing/brainstorming, and (c) leadership and experiential learning. Each of the ten heart-related sessions lasted 90–120 minutes and covered areas such as heart anatomy; risk factors for heart disease, heart attacks, and stroke; diet and exercise; comorbid conditions that affected heart disease risk; and smoking cessation.

Every session began with both informal opportunities for open dialogue and a guided review of information covered in previous sessions. Ongoing discussion incorporated personal experiences and reactions to or recollection of previous sessions. A horseshoe seating arrangement conveyed a sense of visual connectedness and "equality of status" among learners. CHWs completed problem-solving exercises as a large group and in dyads, typically using case scenarios and prepared exercises. These varied from simple exercises to role-playing to opportunities to create new training content. The brainstorming/problem-posing exercises, in contrast, were used to create options for resolving hypothetical and real-life problems. The CHWs had multiple opportunities to lead their peers through sections of the WEHL manual and facilitate exercises. Each CHW was also required to facilitate an abbreviated train-the-trainer session with their peers, incorporating opportunities for group leadership and group facilitation.

The curriculum was adapted to create Web-based learning resources, including brief study guides, audio/video presentations that supported self-directed learning, and access to other educational resources, including electronic versions of the manual and accompanying picture cards. This content, consisting of ten PowerPoint presentations, ten videos, and other text available on the project website and YouTube channel, remained publicly accessible for CHWs to use in facilitating their own CHW trainings and community education sessions.

REFERENCES

Aterman, S., Ghahari, S., & Kessler, D. (2023). Characteristics of peer-based interventions for individuals with neurological conditions: A scoping review. *Disability and Rehabilitation*, 45(2), 344–375. https://doi.org/10.1080/09638288.2022.2028911

Barclay, L., & Hilton, G. M. (2019). A scoping review of peer-led interventions following spinal cord injury. *Spinal Cord*, 57(8), 626–635. https://doi.org/10.1038/s41393-019-0297-x

Beaudoin, M., Best, K. L., & Routhier, F. (2020). Influence of peer-based rehabilitation interventions for improving mobility and participation among adults with mobility disabilities: A systematic review. *Disability and Rehabilitation*, 42(13), 1785–1796. https://doi.org/10.1080/09638288.2018.1537380

Berkanish, P., Pan, S., Viola, A., Rademaker, Q., & Devine, K. A. (2022). Technology-based peer support interventions for adolescents with chronic illness: A systematic review. *Journal of Clinical Psychology in Medical Settings*, 29, 911–942. https://doi.org/10.1007/s10880-022-09853-0

Canter, K. S., & Roberts, M. C. (2012). A systematic and quantitative review of interventions to facilitate school re-entry for children with chronic health conditions. *Journal of Pediatric Psychology*, 37(10), 1065–1075. https://doi.org/10.1093/jpepsy/jss071

Chaffey, L., & Bigby, C. (2018). Health education by peers with spinal cord injury: A scoping review. *Journal of Developmental and Physical Disabilities*, 30, 141–154. https://doi.org/10.1007/s10882-017-9569-6

Clark, E., MacCrosain, A., Ward, N. S., & Jones, F. (2020). The key features and role of peer support within group self-management interventions for stroke: A systematic review. *Disability and Rehabilitation*, 42(3), 307–316. https://doi.org/10.1080/09638288.2018.1498544

Depping, M. K., Uhlenbusch, N., Härter, M., Schramm, C., & Löwe, B. (2021). Efficacy of a brief, peer-delivered self-management intervention for patients with rare chronic diseases: A randomized clinical trial. *JAMA Psychiatry*, 78(6), 607–615. https://doi.org/10.1001/jamapsychiatry.2020.4783

Graham, H., Tokhi, M., & Duke, T. (2016). Scoping review: Strategies of providing care for children with chronic health conditions in low- and middle-income countries. *Tropical Medicine and International Health*, 21(11), 1366–1388. https://doi.org/10.1111/tmi.12774

Hossain, S. N., Jaglal, S. B., Shepherd, J., Perrier, L., Tomasone, J. R., & Sweet, S. N., et al. (2021). Web-based peer support interventions for adults living with chronic conditions: Scoping review. *JMIR Rehabilitation and Assistive Technologies*, 8(2), e14321. https://doi.org/10.2196/14321

Hosseinzadeh, A., Shameli, A., Esmailian, S., & Mohammadnejad, E. (2019). Peer education and heart failure outcome: A review study in Iran. *Iranian Journal of Cardiovascular Nursing, 7*(4), 58–63. https://sid.ir/paper/408715/en

Hughes, R., Fleming, P., & Henshall, L. (2020). Peer support groups after acquired brain injury: A systematic review. *Brain Injury, 34*(7), 847–856. https://doi.org/10.1080/02699052.2020.1762002

Jones, M. J., Gassaway, J., & Sweatman, W. M. (2021). Peer mentoring reduces unplanned readmissions and improves self-efficacy following inpatient rehabilitation for individuals with spinal cord injury. *The Journal of Spinal Cord Medicine, 44*(3), 383–391. https://doi.org/10.1080/10790268.2019.1645407

Karp, N., Yazdany, J., & Schmajuk, G. (2023). Peer support in rheumatic diseases: A narrative literature review. *Patient Preference and Adherence, 17*, 2433–2449. https://doi.org/10.2147/PPA.S391396

Kew, K. M., Carr, R., & Crossingham, I. (2017). Lay-led and peer support interventions for adolescents with asthma. *Cochrane Database of Systematic Reviews, 4*, CD012331. https://doi.org/10.1002/14651858.CD012331.pub2

Kronish, I. M., Goldfinger, J. Z., Negron, R., Fei, K., Tuhrim, S., & Arniella, G., et al. (2014). Effect of peer education on stroke prevention: The prevent recurrence of all inner-city strokes through education randomized controlled trial. *Stroke, 45*(11), 3330–3336. https://doi.org/10.1161/STROKEAHA.114.006623

Levy, B. B., Luong, D., Perrier, L., Bayley, M. T., & Munce, S. E. P. (2019). Peer support interventions for individuals with acquired brain injury, cerebral palsy, and spina bifida: A systematic review. *BMC Health Services Research, 19*(1), 288. https://doi.org/10.1186/s12913-019-4110-5.

Longley, R. M., Harnedy, L. E., Ghanime, P. M., Arroyo-Ariza, D., Deary, E. C., & Daskalakis, E., et al. (2023). Peer support interventions in patients with kidney failure: A systematic review. *Journal of Psychosomatic Research, 171*, 111379. https://doi.org/10.1016/j.jpsychores.2023.111379

Maclachlan, L. R., Mills, K., Lawford, B. J., Egerton, T., Setchell, J., & Hall, L. M., et al. (2020). Design, delivery, maintenance, and outcomes of peer-to-peer online support groups for people with chronic musculoskeletal disorders: Systematic review. *Journal Of Medical Internet Research, 22*(4), e15822. http://www.jmir.org/2020/4/e15822/J

McBrien, K. A., Ivers, N., Barnieh, L., Bailey, J. J., Lorenzetti, D. L., & Nicholas, D., et al. (2018). Patient navigators for people with chronic disease: A systematic review. *PLoS ONE, 13*(2), e0191980. https://doi.org/10.1371/journal.pone.0191980

McIntyre, A., Marrocco, S. L., McRae, S. A., Sleeth, L., Hitzig, S., & Jaglal, S., et al. (2020). A scoping review of self-management interventions following spinal cord injury. *Topics in Spinal Cord Injury Rehabilitation, 26*(1), 36–63. https://doi.org/10.1310/sci2601-36

Merianos, A. L., King, K. A., Vidourek, R. A., & Nabors, L. A. (2016). Mentoring and peer-led interventions to improve quality of life outcomes among adolescents with chronic illnesses. *Applied Research in Quality of Life, 11*, 1009–1023. https://doi.org/10.1007/s11482-015-9415-x

Moore, A., Motagh, S., Sadeghirad, B., Begum, H., Riva, J. J., & Gaber, J., et al. (2021). Volunteer impact on health-related outcomes for seniors: A systematic review and meta-analysis. *Canadian Geriatrics Journal*, 24(1), 44. https://doi.org/10.5770/cgj.24.434

Morris, R. P., Fletcher-Smith, J. C., & Radford, K. A. (2017). A systematic review of peer mentoring interventions for people with traumatic brain injury. *Clinical Rehabilitation*, 31(8), 1030–1038. https://doi.org/10.1177/0269215516676303

Nakao, S., Kamo, T., Someko, H., Okamura, M., Tsujimoto, Y., & Ogihara, H., et al. (2023). Peer support for patients with heart failure: A systematic review and meta-analysis. *Cureus*, 15(10), e46751. https://doi.org/10.7759/cureus.46751

Palacios, J., Lee, G. A., Duaso, M., Clifton, A., Norman, I. J., & Richards, D., et al. (2017). Internet-delivered self-management support for improving coronary heart disease and self-management related outcomes: A systematic review. *Journal of Cardiovascular Nursing*, 32(4), E9–E23. https://doi.org/10.1097/JCN.0000000000000392

Parry, M., & Watt-Watson, J. (2010). Peer support intervention trials for individuals with heart disease: A systematic review. *European Journal of Cardiovascular Nursing*, 9(1), 57–67. https://doi.org/10.1016/j.ejcnurse.2009.10.002

Price, A., de Bell, S., Shaw, N., Bethel, A., Anderson, R., & Coon, J. T. (2022). What is the volume, diversity and nature of recent, robust evidence for the use of peer support in health and social care? An evidence and gap map. *Campbell Systematic Reviews*, 18, e1264. https://doi.org/10.1002/cl2.1264

Rocchi, M. A., Shi, Z. Y., Shaw, R. B., McBride, C. B., & Sweet, S. N. (2022). Identifying the outcomes of participating in peer mentorship for adults living with spinal cord injury: A qualitative meta-synthesis. *Psychology & Health*, 37(4), 523–544. https://www.tandfonline.com/10.1080/08870446.2021.1890729

Runions, K. C., Vithiatharan, R., Hancock, K., Lin, A., Brennan-Jones, C. G., Gray, C., et al. (2020). Chronic health conditions, mental health and the school: A narrative review. *Health Education Journal*, 79(4), 471–483. https://doi.org/10.1177/0017896919890898

Shah, S., Peat, J. K., Mazurski, E. J., Wang, H., Sindhusake, D., & Bruce, C., et al. (2001). Effect of peer led programme for asthma education in adolescents: Cluster randomised controlled trial. *British Medical Journal*, 322(7286), 583. https://doi.org/10.1136/bmj.322.7286.583

Thompson, D. M., Booth, L., Moor, D., & Mathers, J. (2022). Peer support for people with chronic conditions: A systematic review of reviews. *BMC Health Services Research*, 22, 427. https://doi.org/10.1186/s12913-022-07816-7

Wan, X., Chau, J. P. C., Mou, H., & Liu, X. (2021). Effects of peer support interventions on physical and psychosocial outcomes among stroke survivors: A systematic review and meta-analysis. *International Journal of Nursing Studies*, 121, 104001. https://doi.org/10.1016/j.ijnurstu.2021.104001

Wang, F. X., & Guo, L. J. (2019). The study of peer education among discharged patients after mechanical heart valve replacement. *Chinese Journal of Practical Nursing*, 36, 196–200.

Wasilewski, M., Rios, J., Simpson, R., Hitzig, S., Gotlib Conn, L., & MacKay, C., et al. (2023). Peer support for traumatic injury survivors: A scoping review. *Disability and Rehabilitation*, 14(33), 2199–2232. https://doi.org/10.1080/09638288.2022.2083702

Wedege, P., Mæland, S., Abrahamsen, F. E., & Divanoglou, A. (2024). Structured, time-limited peer mentorship activity programmes for individuals with acquired brain or spinal cord injuries: A mixed methods systematic review of characteristics and outcomes. *Disability and Rehabilitation*, *46*, 1–16. https://doi.org/10.1080/09638288.2024.2310185

Willock, R. J., Mayberry, R. M., Yan, F. X., & Daniels, P. (2015). Peer training of community health workers to improve heart health among African American women. *Health Promotion Practice*, *16*(1), 63–71. https://doi.org/10.1177/1524839914535775

Wobma, R., Rinske, H. M. N., Ket, J. C. F., & Kwakkel, G. (2016). Evidence for peer support in rehabilitation for individuals with acquired brain injury: A systematic review. *Journal of Rehabilitation Medicine*, *48*, 837–840. https://doi.org/10.2340/16501977-2160

Zhong, C. S., & Melendez-Torres, G. J. (2017). The effect of peer-led self-management education programmes for adolescents with asthma: A systematic review and meta-analysis. *Health Education Journal*, *76*(6), 676–694. https://doi.org/10.1177/0017896917712297

Mental Health

7

DEFINITION

Poor Mental Health is often associated with stress, anxiety and panic, and sadness and depression. It may stem from feeling lonely or grief after bereavement or loss, or not from any obvious cause, as both life experience and genetic inheritance can be involved in its origin. Suicidal ideation or actual suicide is a risk factor. In its extreme forms (schizophrenia and psychosis), it can be accompanied by paranoia, hallucinations, and hearing voices. Sometimes it is temporary and, in other cases, enduring.

On the other hand, good mental health is more than just the absence of mental illness. Positive mental health is associated with feelings of wellness and resilience to life's mishaps. It means you are in a state of well-being where you feel good and function well in the world. According to the World Health Organisation, good mental health is when you can: cope with the normal stresses of life, learn and work productively, use your talents and abilities, and contribute to the community. If you have good mental health, you might feel happy, confident, hopeful, and generally satisfied with life. You are likely to feel connected to other people. You might also have a sense of meaning or purpose and a feeling of being at peace.

Specific mental health disorders include Agoraphobia, Anorexia nervosa, Antisocial personality disorder, Binge eating disorder, Bipolar disorder, Body dysmorphic disorder, Borderline personality disorder, Bulimia, Claustrophobia, Cyclothymia, Dissociative disorders, Eating disorders, Health anxiety, Hoarding disorder, Munchausen syndrome, Obsessive-Compulsive disorder (OCD), Panic disorder, Personality disorder, Phobias, Postpartum psychosis, Post-traumatic stress disorder (PTSD), Psychosis, Schizophrenia, Seasonal affective disorder (SAD), Selective mutism, Skin picking disorder and Trichotillomania (hair pulling disorder). If necessary, look them up on the internet.

DOI: 10.1201/9781003438366-7   91

REVIEWS OF EVIDENCE

There were 40 reviews of evidence. The great majority were on mental health in general, some with an emphasis on adolescents/youth and schools/universities.

Five focused on depression including, suicide prevention, and one on schizophrenia.

General Mental Health

Repper and Carter (2010) searched three databases from 1995 to 2010. However, only seven Randomized Controlled Trials (RCTs) met the inclusion criteria, and they had inconsistent findings. According to Davidson et al. (2012), peers could be effective in engaging people into care, reducing the use of emergency rooms and hospitals, and reducing substance use among persons with co-occurring substance use disorders. When providing peer support that involves positive self-disclosure, role modeling, and conditional regard, peer staff also increased participants' sense of hope, control, and ability to effect changes in their lives; increased their self-care, sense of community belonging, and satisfaction with various life domains; and decreased participants' level of depression and psychosis. Miyamoto and Sono (2012) included 51 studies, including eight review articles and 19 qualitative studies. Most of the challenges concerned how peer supporters related to people receiving peer support and how peer support providers were treated in the system.

Lloyd-Evans et al. (2014) searched five databases in 2013 and included 18 trials: four trials of mutual support programs, eleven trials of peer support services, and three trials of peer-delivered services. There was some evidence that peer support was associated with positive effects on measures of hope, recovery, and empowerment at and beyond the end of the intervention. However, there were no effects on hospitalization. A systematic review was conducted by Campos et al. (2014), searching four databases from 2001 to 2013 and including 112 documents, identifying as main peer support categories: characterization, peer supporter, practices, and efficacy. However, findings were mixed. Chinman et al. (2014) searched eight databases from 1995 to 2012 and identified 20 studies. A majority of studies of two service types – peers added and peers delivering curricula – showed some improvement favoring peers. Compared with professional staff, peers were better able to reduce in-patient use and improve a range of recovery outcomes. A systematic review by Stubbs et al. (2016) investigated peers seeking to improve physical health, lifestyle, or physical health appointment attendance in participants with severe mental illness. Seven articles were included, including three RCTs. Three studies found that peer support had resulted in small reductions in weight. Only one study demonstrated that peer support improved self-reported physical activity and diet. Evidence regarding physical health appointment attendance was also unclear across four studies.

Payne (2017) commented on peer support as relevant to social work practice. Employing peers as supporters for people recovering from mental ill-health was feasible both in peer-led and professional mental health provision. Outcomes were at least as good as professional help, and peer support reduced the use of expensive in-patient services. Meta-analyses and systematic reviews were searched for by Bellamy et al. (2017), who also found individual studies not included in any of the reviews. Peer services were generally equally effective to services provided by non-peer paraprofessionals on traditional clinical outcomes. Some studies found peer services effective at reducing hospitalization rates and symptom severity. Peer support had a positive impact on levels of hope, empowerment, and quality of life. Only one study had a negative finding. Villani and Kovess-Masféty (2018) noted that the therapeutic efficiency of peer support had been proven by several controlled studies as being at least as good as traditional services and even better in some specific areas. Their review investigated the situation in France in comparison with other countries, searching seven databases from 2005 to 2016 and including 32 papers. There was evidence of many benefits for service users such as the optional aspect of this care process, a more authentic therapeutic relationship, a less normative frame, an active partnership, and a more optimistic philosophy aiming to make "small steps" toward improvement. Health professionals and peer supporters themselves had found benefits during the process.

Quantitative evidence was synthesized by Burke et al. (2019), who searched seven databases in 2017 and included 23 studies: peer-led group interventions, one-to-one peer support, and peer-run services. Results suggested that peer-facilitated time-limited group interventions could result in small but significant improvements in empowerment and self-efficacy compared with treatment as usual. Evidence was inconclusive for one-to-one peer support, peer-run services, and internalized stigma. Shalaby and Agyapong (2020) searched six databases. There was an international trend to adopt peer support within addiction and mental health services, and despite challenges, much of the current literature supported the inclusion of peer support workers in the mental health care workforce. Four databases were searched by Shin and Choi (2020), and 14 studies were included in a systematic review, including eight RCTs. Overall, peer support was found effective in reducing hospitalization rates, hospitalization days, the number of emergency room visits, and total medical costs. The evidence that peer support was associated with positive effects on measures of psychiatric symptoms, quality of life, and social support was inconsistent.

A focus on one-to-one peer support by White et al. (2020) on 11 studies yielded evidence that one-to-one peer support had a modest positive impact on self-reported recovery and empowerment. However, there was no impact on clinical symptoms or service use. Peer support might improve social network support. Fortuna et al. (2020) reviewed peer-supported digital interventions, searching seven databases from 1946 to 2018 and including 30 studies (11 RCTs) reporting 24 interventions. Most of the studies demonstrated the feasibility, acceptability, and effectiveness of peer-to-peer networks, peer-delivered interventions supported with technology, and the use of asynchronous and synchronous technologies. The impact of the COVID pandemic on mental health and the utility of peer support in combating this 2019–2021 was studied by Suresh et al. (2021). Three databases were searched. The pandemic had ubiquitously worsened mental health across the world. Peer support has been demonstrated to yield generally positive effects on the mental health of a wide variety of recipients, although there were a few conflicting studies.

Mutschler et al. (2022) synthesized the literature on the implementation of peer support interventions. The systematic search identified 19 articles and highlighted important elements for implementation, including clear role definition, a flexible organizational culture, and education for both peer and non-peer staff. Five databases were searched by Høgh et al. (2023) for RCTs, leading to a meta-analysis including 49 studies, many with high risk of bias. Peer support had a small positive effect on personal recovery (effect size = 0.20) and decreased anxiety symptoms (effect size = 0.21). There was a modest effect on self-advocacy. Searches in three databases to 2020 were conducted by Smit et al. (2023), including 30 RCTs in a systematic review. Peer support was associated with small but significant post-test effect sizes for clinical recovery (g = 0.19) and personal recovery (g = 0.15), but not for functional recovery (g = 0.08). Effects were modest but consistent, suggesting efficacy across a wide range of mental disorders and intervention types.

Cooper et al. (2024) searched five databases from 2012 to 2022 for reviews of paid peer support interventions, including 35 reviews of which 23 investigated effectiveness. Results were mixed. There was some evidence from meta-analyses that peer support might improve depression symptoms (particularly perinatal depression), self-efficacy, and recovery. Factors promoting successful implementation included adequate training and supervision, a recovery-oriented workplace, strong leadership, and a supportive and trusting workplace culture with effective collaboration. Peer support could bring recovery and improved well-being, but there was sometimes confusion over the peer supporter role and organizational challenges, including low pay, negative non-peer staff attitudes, and lack of support and training. Five databases from 2005 to 2022 were searched by Murphy et al. (2024), who included 15 studies. The review supported previous research indicating that peer support had potential for improving recovery-related outcomes. Examples of barriers to implementation included staff concerns around confidentiality of peer support relationships as well as supporters' confidence in their roles.

Depression (Including Perinatal Depression) and Suicide

Melling and Houguet-Pincham (2011) searched published literature on online peer support services for people with depression, which had many potential advantages. However, there was limited empirical evidence of the efficacy of such services. In the same year, Pfeiffer et al. (2011) identified seven RCTs of peer support versus usual care for depression. Peer support interventions were superior to usual care in reducing depressive symptoms, with an average effect size of 0.59 (p = 0.002).

McLeish et al. (2023) focused on perinatal depression, including 29 studies of 22 interventions offering support by one-to-one or group peer support, in person or by telephone. Positive impact was noted in receiving empathetic listening, acceptance, affirmation, and normalization; peers sharing ideas about self-care, coping, and services; peers using therapeutic techniques; the opportunity to give support to others; and meaningful social relationships with volunteers and other mothers. Negative impact concerned self-criticism from downward and upward social comparison; peers being judgmental or directive; not feeling heard; peer support could be a stressful social relationship; and distress at endings. Perinatal depression was also the focus of Liblub et al. (2024), who sought insights into evidence on mobile health and peer support. A scoping review of five databases from 2007 to 2022 led to the inclusion of eight studies. Results showed decreased depressive scores. Strong satisfaction with the accessibility and flexibility of mobile health was found when combined with peer support.

Hildebrand et al. (2019) noted suicide was the second most prevalent cause of death among 15–25-year-olds worldwide, and identified online peer counselling services for suicide prevention in youth and young adults. Thirteen studies were included. Generally, the literature showed positive results concerning implementation, satisfaction, and efficacy. However, many studies exhibited methodological deficiencies.

Schizophrenia

Evans (2023) conducted a systematic scoping review on peer support reaching people with schizophrenia that included 22 studies describing 20 interventions. Three of four studies that measured negative symptoms reported significant changes favoring peer services. Results were mixed but a study of peer-led mutual support groups for people with schizophrenia and their families in China demonstrated favorable outcomes over three years in overall functioning and reductions in duration and number of hospitalizations. Mutual support groups for adults with psychotic disorders in the Netherlands demonstrated positive effects on contact with peers outside of sessions and esteem support. High attenders showed significant improvements in social support, self-efficacy, and quality of life compared to low attenders. In a study of telephone-based peer support for people with schizophrenia in Australia, participants improved in medication adherence and total symptoms over a period of 14 weeks and reduced negative symptoms.

Youth and Adolescence

Ali et al. (2015) noted adolescence was a critical period for the development of mental disorders and offered a systematic review of online peer-to-peer support. Three databases were searched and six studies were included. Four studies investigated Internet support groups and two focused on virtual reality chat sessions. Two of the three RCTs were associated with a significant positive outcome in comparison to the control group at post-intervention. In the remaining studies, peer support was not effective. A literature review of peer support for young people (of school age) was conducted by Coleman et al. (2017) for 2006–2016. Peer support schemes differed in source of delivery, approach or activities, and aims. Models included school-based one-to-one support and school-based group support, all involving structured training for supporters. Peer support schemes could also be online, which could offer a degree of anonymity to participants. There were also community-based projects run by voluntary organizations. In general, the evidence on effectiveness could be divided between a small number of studies including robust evaluations; and a larger number of studies based on feedback from participants and self-reported outcomes, such as increased happiness and wellbeing, improved self-esteem, confidence, and emotional resilience, improved social skills and relationships, and positive impact on the school environment. Many studies also noted the positive effect for peer supporters. Several studies noted the importance of the program being well run, with a clear focus, strong leadership, and support throughout the school. A number of studies stressed the value of co-production of schemes by children or young people. Specific key elements included: a structured process of monitoring and evaluation; having a dedicated space for peer support, with dedicated time slots; and formal training of peer supporters and coordinators.

Richard et al. (2022) searched seven databases and included 17 studies. Overall, they suggested that peer support was associated with improvements in mental health, including greater happiness, self-esteem, and effective coping, and reductions in depression, loneliness, and anxiety. This was the case with university students, non-student young adults, and ethnic/sexual minorities. Both individual and group peer support appeared to be beneficial, with positive effects also for those providing the support. The effectiveness of peer support for youth depression and anxiety was investigated by Simmons et al. (2023), searching four databases from 1980 to 2022. Nine RCTs were included, seven in high-income countries. One study successfully reduced anxiety and depression, another reduced depression only, four reported reductions in negative affect, with the final three not having a significant impact on depression.

Schools and Universities

John et al. (2018) reviewed the evidence for the effectiveness of peer support in improving mental health well-being in university students, searching six electronic databases. However, only three studies met the inclusion criteria, one of which found social support to be the most important protective factor for mental well-being, while two showed no statistically significant improvement. A systematic review by King and Fazel (2021) searched 11 databases and included 11 studies. Two studies out of five that looked at peer recipient outcomes showed significant improvements in self-confidence and in a quality-of-life measure. Peer leaders showed significant improvements in self-esteem and social stress, with one study showing an increase in guilt. Pointon-Haas et al. (2023) investigated peer support in universities, searching five databases and including 28 papers. The heterogeneity of measures and outcomes prevented firm conclusions on the effectiveness of peer support for mental health and well-being.

Vocational Groups

Ho et al. (2022) studied migrant domestic workers, searching eight databases and including 12 articles. Two types of peer support were identified: mutual aid and trained peer support. Mutual aid was mainly for emotional comfort, while the peer support training program was highly culturally appropriate. However, there were concerns about emotion contagion among peers, worries about the disclosure of personal information, and lack of support from health professionals. Public safety workers were studied by Fallon et al. (2023), including correctional officers, law enforcement, firefighters, emergency medical service, and military personnel. Exposure to traumatic events, job hazards, injuries, fatalities, and stressors such as work overload, irregular shift assignments, and lack of administrative support could be problematic. A scoping review was conducted in six databases from 1996 to 2021, and 13 articles were included. Organizational support, including policies, practices, and peer leadership training, contributed to the sustainability of peer support. Confidentiality, trust, and shared lived experience were also essential. Participants found peer support helpful in normalizing experiences, increasing hope, and decreasing stigma.

Peer Supporters

Walker and Bryant (2013) investigated 27 qualitative studies. Peer support workers experiences included staff discrimination and prejudice, low pay, and difficulty managing the transition from "patient" to peer supporter. Positive experiences included collegial relationships with staff and other peers, and increased wellness. Structurally embedding peer supporters in practice can be challenging, as De Beer et al. (2022) noted. A total of 24 studies were included, and six roles and five themes were identified. Roles included the engagement role, emotional support role, navigating and planning role, advocacy role, research role, and the educational role. The themes concerned the needs of peer supporters, their experiences, relationships between service users and peer supporters, the collaboration process with non-peer staff, and organizational readiness. Peer support requires careful planning.

SINGLE STUDIES

Number of Single Studies

There were 81 individual studies. Of these, 59 concerned general Mental Health and nine with Depression. Autism, Bullying, Eating Disorders, Schizophrenia, and Suicide Prevention all had two papers. Single papers dealt with Anxiety, Hypertension, Self-injury, and OCDs. Only five papers (out of 81, 6%) were from developing countries, with a further four targeting minority populations in developed countries. As the literature reviews were so numerous, only two single studies from each of the developed and developing countries will be described here.

Exemplar Single Studies Developed Context

Cheng and Yen (2021) located peer support within vocational services for persons with schizophrenia. Six peers were willing and were trained to co-lead workplace problem-solving groups and care skills training in an extended vocational rehabilitation program. The social support, mental health, psychiatric symptoms, and functioning of service users were assessed before and after peer-delivered services. Assessments were based on the Social Support Scale (SSS), Chinese Health Questionnaire-12 (CHQ-12), Brief Psychiatric Rating Scale (BPRS), Global Assessment of Function (GAF), and the Chinese version of the Social Functioning Scale (C-SFS). The recruited 46 service users were mostly middle-aged (mean age 49), with 27 being male (59%). After interventions, the 42 service users who completed the program had a significantly increased SSS score (p = 0.01). The objective (p = 0.001) and subjective (p = 0.01) social functional scores both significantly increased. The weekly wage elevated significantly (p = 0.01) and the BPRS-18 score decreased significantly (p = 0.007). Peer-delivered vocational rehabilitation services may enhance the social support received by persons with schizophrenia and improve their occupational outcomes.

In a pilot program, Drouin et al. (2023) developed a peer support network to address multi-morbidity involving intimate partner violence, suicidal ideation, and depression. The peer supporters were termed Suicide Obviation Support (SOS) navigators. The SOS navigators provided direct support and continuity of care for these high-risk patients, which included referrals to mental health treatment and other types of support services, such as transportation and emergency housing. Over one year, support was given to 108 patients (68% women) who screened positive for intimate partner violence, many of whom also screened at moderate or high risk for suicidality (65%) and/or exhibited depression symptoms. At six-month follow-up, 63 participants (58%) were retained. Those who stayed enrolled in the program for six months were less likely to report partner violence and depression symptoms and were at a lower risk for suicide than the original sample. Partner violence, depression, and suicide risk scores declined significantly in this group. This program provided a model for peer support programs for individuals facing multiple, acute mental health care needs.

Exemplar Single Studies Developing Context

Murphy et al. (2017) conducted a reciprocal peer education program focused on problem-based learning between medical students in the UK and in Somaliland, using a program developed by the World Health Organisation. Twelve pairs of UK and Somaliland medical students completed the full program. Participants met online at their mutual convenience via the low-bandwidth Medicine Africa website for problem-based tutorials focused on modules of the program. Pre- and post-participation surveys were used for evaluation. Median scores for Somaliland ($p = 0.003$) and UK students ($p = 0.011$) improved significantly. Qualitative feedback showed that participants valued peer connectivity and learning about cultural and psychosocial differences in their partner's country. Somaliland students were motivated by clinical learning and UK students by global health education. Feedback on the problem-based learning structure was positive. Digital problem-based learning represented an innovative method to extend the benefits of learning beyond front-line clinical staff to healthcare students. Educational resource limitations in low- and middle-income countries could be overcome in this way.

In Iran, Daryadokht et al. (2017) investigated the effect of peer education on the adherence to prescribed drugs and the quality of life of hypertensive patients in two hospitals – 55 cases were selected for both intervention and control groups. Data collection tools included three questionnaires: demographic, medication adherence, and quality of life (with 36 questions on eight dimensions: general health, physical functioning, role-playing limitations due to physical problems, role-playing limitations due to emotional problems, somatic pain, social functioning, fatigue, and mental health or vitality). The intervention patients experienced training from trained peers during three one-hour sessions over three days. The peers shared their experiences on how to control the disease in the patients by collaborating with each other. The control group underwent routine training by a physician using posters in the clinics. Pre-intervention, participants in both control and intervention groups had poor adherence to drugs. The changes in adherence to the drugs in the intervention group showed that the average adherence in the intervention group increased after the intervention, but in the control group, it decreased ($p = 0.001$). There was also a significant relationship between peer education and quality of life.

SPECIFIC PROGRAM

The specific program was located in South Africa (Swartz et al., 2012).

Effectiveness

This paper reports an evaluation of a peer-led intervention, entitled Vhutshilo, implemented by the Harvard School of Public Health and the Centre for the Support of Peer Education (the Rutanang collaboration). Vhutshilo targeted vulnerable adolescents aged 14–16 years living in some of South Africa's under-resourced communities. Vhutshilo programs for this age group were implemented at 11 sites in Gauteng and Limpopo. There were 73 participants (43 girls and 30 boys) in the intervention group and 110 (75 girls and 35 boys) in the control (wait-list) group. Questionnaires were administered twice for recipients of peer education ($n = 73$), immediately after completion of the program (post-test) and four months later (delayed post-test), and once for control group members ($n = 110$). Semi-structured interviews ($n = 32$) were also conducted with recipients of peer education. Survey questionnaires were administered in respondents' language of choice, although most chose to complete the English version, using the vernacular versions as a reference. A fieldworker was in the room during survey completion, and answered questions of clarity. Six statistically significant changes were observed in Vhutshilo participants.

Youth struggling with poor quality education and living in economically fraught contexts with little social support, nonetheless, showed evidence of having greater knowledge of support networks and an expanded emotional repertoire by the end of the Vhutshilo program, and four months later. Results regarding the relationship between SES and peer education suggested that extremely low socio-economic status (SES) may weaken the effectiveness of peer education, while marginally higher SES may promote its effectiveness. Nonetheless, many participants with low SES showed great improvement with regard to program indicator scores. When well organized and properly supported the Vhutshilo curriculum provided vulnerable youth with opportunities to develop psychosocial skills and informational resources that contributed to the changing of norms, attitudes, and behaviors.

Implementation

In the South African context, the pervasive effect of poverty means that many young people have limited assets with which to develop resilience to environmental threats and risky health and social behaviors. Poverty, when combined with the usual social upheavals of adolescence, renders interventions crucial for the youth. These interventions need to address social and behavioral factors that impact adolescents' risk-taking, and should bolster their psychosocial capacities to deal with poverty and vulnerability. These negative social and behavioral factors include alcohol and drug use; participation in and exposure to crime and violence; involvement in transactional sex, unprotected sex, inter-generational sexual relationships, and multiple concurrent partnerships; high school dropout and subsequent unemployment as a result of teenage pregnancy and inadequate access to public health facilities by young people. In South Africa, the school dropout rate increases dramatically after Grade 9. School dropout, in turn, is highly correlated to teenage pregnancy among females and teenage fatherhood among males.

The paper reports an evaluation of a peer education program entitled Vhutshilo (meaning 'Life' in Venda) carried out by the Human Sciences Research Council (HSRC) of South Africa. The focus was on the program's effects on youth participants and on the methodology used in the evaluation. The impact of peer education extended from building self-esteem to motivating youth to address challenges, to promoting academic performance and positively influencing behavior. Vhutshilo is a curriculum-based peer education program for adolescents designed by the Harvard School of Public Health and its South African Centre for the Support of Peer Education, with financial backing from the US President's Emergency Plan for AIDS Relief. The program serves 14–16-year-olds and is facilitated by 17–19-year-olds. It sought to encourage learning that could not be achieved in other settings, such as the classroom or at home, to develop the knowledge, attitudes, beliefs, and life skills required for youth to engage in healthy behaviors.

The program consisted of 13 one-hour sessions, with sequential learning objectives and participatory methods specifically developed for peer delivery in after-school settings. Illustrations and real-life scenarios encouraged participants to think and talk with each other. Vhutshilo followed a cast of characters and a storyline that was sustained throughout the sessions, using visual cartoon characters. The program helped adolescent participants to express and cope with feelings of loss and grief, and to identify services, people, and places in their community that provided help. In emphasizing age-appropriate prevention strategies, Vhutshilo stressed healthy adolescent development, healthy relationships, awareness of the threats posed by inter-generational and transactional sex, and the dangers of multiple concurrent partnerships. Vhutshilo was designed to be a practical intervention that could be implemented at scale under real-world conditions. It relied on effective adult supervision through appropriate selection, training, and support of on-site supervisors from partner organizations, who in turn recruited, trained, and supervised peer educators. The approach informing the Vhutshilo curriculum was derived through a national consultative process, which developed rigorous field standards and a comprehensive training and support strategy for South African peer education programs. These are described at length in the Rutanang documents that emerged from this process (see original paper for references).

Rutanang (meaning 'Learning from One Another') provided multiple standards that required peer education programs to devote adequate attention to:

1. Planning and mobilizing a system in which peer education occurs, with linkages for follow-up and referral;
2. Developing an adult infrastructure of training and support, alongside a cohort of trained and supported peer educators;
3. Devising a learning program and pedagogical frame;
4. Managing and rewarding performance; and
5. Monitoring and evaluating inputs and impact.

Furthermore, Rutanang posited four roles for peer educators, who were trained and assisted by adult supervisors. These were to:

1. Educate their peers in a structured manner;
2. Informally role-model healthy behavior;
3. Recognize youth in need of additional help and refer them for assistance; and
4. Advocate for resources and services for themselves and their peers.

Rutanang standards were integral to both the design of Vhutshilo and its evaluation.

REFERENCES

Ali, K., Farrer, L., Gulliver, A., & Griffiths, K. M. (2015). Online peer-to-peer support for young people with mental health problems: A systematic review. *JMIR Mental Health*, *2*(2), e19. https://doi.org/10.2196/mental.4418

Bellamy, C., Schmutte, T., & Davidson, L. (2017). An update on the growing evidence base for peer support. *Mental Health and Social Inclusion*, *21*(3), 1–7. https://doi.org/10.1108/MHSI-03-2017-0014

Burke, E., Pyle, M., Machin, K., Varese, F., & Morrison, A. P. (2019). The effects of peer support on empowerment, self-efficacy, and internalized stigma: A narrative synthesis and meta-analysis. *Stigma and Health*, *4*(3), 337–356. https://doi.org/10.1037/sah0000148

Campos, F. A. L., de Sousa, A. R. P., da Costa Rodrigues, V. P., da Silva Marques, A. J. P., da Rocha Dores, A. A. M., & Queirós, C. M. L. (2014). Peer support for people with mental illness. *Revista De Psiquiatria Clínica*, *41*(2), 49–55. https://doi.org/10.1590/0101-60830000000009

Cheng, K. Y., & Yen, C. F. (2021). The social support, mental health, psychiatric symptoms, and functioning of persons with schizophrenia participating in peer co-delivered vocational rehabilitation: a pilot study in Taiwan. *BMC psychiatry*, *21*(1), 268. https://doi.org/10.1186/s12888-021-03277-0

Chinman, M., Preethy, G., Dougherty, R. D., Daniels, A. S., Ghose, S. S., & Swift, A., et al. (2014). Peer support services for individuals with serious mental illnesses: Assessing the evidence. *Psychiatric Services*, *65*, 429–441. https://doi.org/10.1176/appi.ps.201300244

Coleman, N., Sykes, W., & Groom, C. (2017). *Peer support and children and young people's mental health*. London: Department for Education.

Cooper, R. E., Saunders, K. R. K., Greenburgh, A., Shah, P., Appleton, R., & Machin, K., et al. (2024). The effectiveness, implementation, and experiences of peer support approaches for mental health: A systematic umbrella review. *BMC Medicine*, *22*(1), 72. https://doi.org/10.1186/s12916-024-03260-y

Daryadokht, M. R., Elahe, M. B., & Hamid, H. (2017). Effect of peer education on the medication adherence and the quality of life of hypertensive patients. *Pharmacophore*, *8*(3), 19–23.

Davidson, L., Bellamy, C., Guy, K., & Miller, R. (2012). Peer support among persons with severe mental illnesses: A review of evidence and experience. *World Psychiatry*, *11*(2), 123–128. https://doi.org/10.1016/j.wpsyc.2012.05.009

de Beer, C. R. M., Nooteboom, L. A., van Domburgh, L., de Vreugd, M., Schoones, J. W., & Vermeiren, R. R. J. M. (2022). A systematic review exploring youth peer support for young people with mental health problems. *European Child & Adolescent Psychiatry*, 1–14. https://doi.org/10.1007/s00787-022-02120-5

Drouin, M., Flanagan, M., Carroll, J., Kerrigan, C., Henry, H., & Toscos, T. (2023). Piloting a peer support program for patients who screen positive for intimate partner violence, suicidal ideation, and depression. *Healthcare*, *11*(17), 2422. https://doi.org/10.3390/healthcare11172422

Evans, M. (2023). *Peer support services reaching people with schizophrenia*. Cham, Switzerland: Springer. https://doi.org/10.1007/978-3-031-29042-8.

Fallon, P., Jaegers, L. A., Zhang, Y., Dugan, A. G., Cherniack, M., & El Ghaziri, M. (2023). Peer support programs to reduce organizational stress and trauma for public safety workers: A scoping review. *Workplace Health & Safety*, *71*(11), 523–535. https://doi.org/10.1177/21650799231194623

Fortuna, K. L., Naslund, J. A., LaCroix, J. M., Bianco, C. L., Brooks, J. M., & Zisman-Ilani, Y., et al. (2020). Digital peer support mental health interventions for people with a lived experience of a serious mental illness: Systematic review. *JMIR Mental Health*, *7*(4), e16460. https://doi.org/10.2196/16460

Hildebrand, A., Weiss, M., & Stemmler, M. (2019). Online peer-to-peer suicide prevention programs in youth and young adults: A systematic review. *Zeitschrift fur Psychiatrie Psychologie Und Psychotherapie*, *67*(4), 221–229.

Høgh, E. C., Heinsvig, P. C., Hjorthøj, C., Skriver, M. S., Hellström, L., & Nørgaard, N. M.; et al. (2023). The effectiveness of peer support in personal and clinical recovery: Systematic review and meta-analysis. *Psychiatric Services*, *74*(8), 847–858. https://doi.org/10.1176/appi.ps.202100138

Ho, K. H. M., Yang, C., Leung, A. K. Y., Bressington, D., Chien, W. T., & Cheng, Q., et al. (2022). Peer SUPPORT and mental health of migrant domestic workers: A scoping review. *International Journal of Environmental Research and Public Health*, *19*(13). https://doi.org/10.3390/ijerph19137617

John, N. M., Page, O., Martin, S. C., & Whittaker, P. (2018). Impact of peer support on student mental wellbeing: A systematic review. *MedEdPublish*, *7*, 170. https://doi.org/10.15694/mep.2018.0000170.1

King, T., & Fazel, M. (2021). Examining the mental health outcomes of school-based peer-led interventions on young people: A scoping review of range and a systematic review of effectiveness. *PLoS ONE*, *16*(4), e0249553. https://doi.org/10.1371/journal.pone.0249553

Liblub, S., Pringle, K., McLaughlin, K., & Cummins, A. (2024). Peer support and Mobile health for perinatal mental health: A scoping review. *Birth*, *51*(3), 484–496. https://doi.org/10.1111/birt.12814

Lloyd-Evans, B., Mayo-Wilson, E., Harrison, B., Istead, H., Brown, E., & Pilling, S., et al. (2014). A systematic review and meta-analysis of randomised controlled trials of peer support for people with severe mental illness. *BMC Psychiatry*, *14*, 39. http://www.biomedcentral.com/1471-244X/14/39

McLeish, J., Ayers, S., & McCourt, C. (2023). Community-based perinatal mental health peer support: A realist review. *BMC Pregnancy and Childbirth*, *23*(1), 570. https://doi.org/10.1186/s12884-023-05843-8

Melling, B., & Houguet-Pincham, T. (2011). Online peer support for individuals with depression: A summary of current research and future considerations. *Psychiatric Rehabilitation Journal*, *34*(3), 252–254. https://doi.org/10.2975/34.3.2011.252.254

Miyamoto, Y., & Sono, T. (2012). Lessons from peer support among individuals with mental health difficulties: A review of the literature. *Clinical Practice & Epidemiology in Mental Health*, *8*, 22–29. https://doi.org/10.2174/1745017901208010022

Murphy, R., Clissold, E., & Keynejad, R. C. (2017). Problem-based, peer-to-peer global mental health e-learning between the UK and somaliland: A pilot study. *Evidence-Based Mental Health*, *20*(4), 142–146. https://doi.org/10.1136/eb-2017-102766

Murphy, R., Huggard, L., Fitzgerald, A., Hennessy, E., & Booth, A. (2024). A systematic scoping review of peer support interventions in integrated primary youth mental health care. *Journal of Community Psychology*, *52*(1), 154–180.

Mutschler, C., Bellamy, C., Davidson, L., Lichtenstein, S., & Kidd, S. (2022). Implementation of peer support in mental health services: A systematic review of the literature. *Psychological Services*, *19*(2), 360–374. https://doi.org/10.1037/ser0000531

Payne, M. (2017). Peer support in mental health: A narrative review of its relevance to social work. *The Egyptian Journal of Social Work*, *4*(1), 19–40. https://doi.org/10.21608/EJSW.2017.8725

Pfeiffer, P. N., Heisler, M., Piette, J. D., Rogers, M. A., & Valenstein, M. (2011). Efficacy of peer support interventions for depression: A meta-analysis. *General Hospital Psychiatry*, *33*(1), 29–36. https://doi.org/10.1016/j.genhosppsych.2010.10.002

Pointon-Haas, J., Waqar, L., Upsher, R., Foster, J., Byrom, N., & Oates, J. (2023). A systematic review of peer support interventions for student mental health and well-being in higher education. *British Journal of Psychiatry*, *10*(1), e12. https://doi.org/10.1192/bjo.2023.603

Repper, J., & Carter, T. (2010). *Using personal experience to support others with similar difficulties: A review of the literature on peer support in mental health services.* London: Together-UK.

Richard, J., Rebinsky, R., Suresh, R., Kubic, S., Carter, A., & Cunningham, J. E. A., et al. (2022). Scoping review to evaluate the effects of peer support on the mental health of young adults. *BMJ Open, 12,* e061336. https://doi.org/10.1136/bmjopen-2022-061336

Shalaby, R. A. H., & Agyapong, V. I. O. (2020). Peer Support in mental health: Literature review. *JMIR Mental Health, 7(6),* e15572. https://doi.org/10.2196/15572

Shin, S. Y., & Choi, H. S. (2020). A systematic review on peer support services related to the mental health services utilization for people with severe mental illness. *Journal of Korean Academy of Psychiatric and Mental Health Nursing, 29(1),* 51–63. https://doi.org/10.12934/jkpmhn.2020.29.1.51

Simmons, M. B., Cartner, S., MacDonald, R., Whitson, S., Bailey, A., & Brown, E. (2023). The effectiveness of peer support from a person with lived experience of mental health challenges for young people with anxiety and depression: A systematic review. *BMC Psychiatry, 23,* 194. https://doi.org/10.1186/s12888-023-04578-2

Smit, D., Miguel, C., Vrijsen, J. N., Groeneweg, B., Spijker, J., & Cuijpers, P. (2023). The effectiveness of peer support for individuals with mental illness: Systematic review and meta-analysis. *Psychological Medicine, 53,* 5332–5341. https://doi.org/10.1017/S0033291722002422

Stubbs, B., Williams, J., Shannon, J., Gaughran, F., & Craig, T. (2016). Peer support interventions seeking to improve physical health and lifestyle behaviours among people with serious mental illness: A systematic review. *International Journal of Mental Health Nursing, 25(6),* 484–495. https://doi.org/10.1111/inm.12256.

Suresh, R., Alam, A., & Karkossa, Z. (2021). Using peer support to strengthen mental health during the COVID-19 pandemic: A review. *Frontiers in Psychiatry, 12,* 714181. https://doi.org/10.3389/fpsyt.2021.714181

Swartz, S., Deutsch, C., Makoae, M., Michel, B., Harding, J. H., & Garzouzie, G., et al. (2012). Measuring change in vulnerable adolescents: Findings from a peer education evaluation in South Africa. *Journal of Social Aspects of HIV/AIDS, 9(4),* 241–254.

Villani, M., & Kovess-Masféty, V. (2018). Peer support programs in mental health in France: Status report and challenges. *L'Encephale, 44(5),* 457–464. https://doi.org/10.1016/j.encep.2018.01.003

Walker, G., & Bryant, W. (2013). Peer support in adult mental health services: A metasynthesis of qualitative findings. *Psychiatric Rehabilitation Journal, 36(1),* 28–34. https://doi.org/10.1037/h0094744

White, S., Foster, R., & Marks, J. *et al.* (2020). The effectiveness of one-to-one peer support in mental health services: A systematic review and meta-analysis. *BMC Psychiatry,* 20, 534. https://doi.org/10.1186/s12888-020-02923-3

Alcohol Abuse

8

DEFINITION

Alcohol, sometimes referred to as ethanol, is a psychoactive depressant drug that is the active ingredient in fermented drinks such as beer, wine, and distilled spirits. Alcohol produces happiness and euphoria, decreased anxiety, increased sociability, sedation, impairment of cognitive, memory, motor, and sensory function, and generalized depression of the central nervous system. Alcohol has been used for a great many years. Beer was likely brewed from barley as early as 11,000 BC in the Middle East. Alcohol was brewed in 7,000 BC in northern China. The earliest evidence of winemaking was in 6,000 BC in Georgia. Consequently, it is more widely socially acceptable than other drugs, and this is perhaps reflected in the small number of relevant studies.

Short-term adverse effects include generalized impairment of neurocognitive function, dizziness, nausea, vomiting, and hangover-like symptoms. Alcohol is addictive and can result in alcohol use disorder, dependence, and withdrawal. It can have a variety of long-term adverse effects on health, such as liver cirrhosis, brain damage, some cancers, and cardiovascular diseases. Alcoholism refers to alcohol addiction and alcohol dependence. Alcohol dependence is linked to a lifespan that is reduced by about 12 years relative to the average person.

Alcohol consumption by an expectant mother may cause fetal alcohol syndrome and pre-term birth complications. Alcohol can also result in harm to other people, such as family members, friends, co-workers, and strangers. A significant proportion of problems from alcohol consumption arises from unintentional and intentional injuries, including those due to road traffic crashes, violence, and suicide, which tend to occur in relatively younger age groups. The percentage of alcohol-attributable deaths among men amounts to 7.7% of all global deaths compared to 2.6% of all deaths among women.

REVIEWS OF EVIDENCE

There were six reviews which included peer education, counseling, or support, but only half focused wholly on this topic, and two of these were with university/college students. Turning to the mixed studies first, a systematic review and meta-analysis on peer-led interventions to prevent tobacco, alcohol and/or drug use among young people aged 11–21 years was reported by MacArthur, et al. (2015). Only randomized controlled trials (RCTs) were included, and 17 eligible studies were found. However, only six studies representing 1,699 individuals in 66 schools demonstrated that peer-led interventions were associated with benefits in relation to alcohol use (ES = 0.80, p = 0.036), albeit with a substantial effect size.

Peer-delivered services for substance abuse in low- and middle-income countries were systematically reviewed by Satinsky et al. (2021), who searched four international and six region-specific databases and included 34 articles. Some of these articles demonstrated positive impacts of peer-delivered services, including reductions in risk behaviors, but many others showed no significant difference in outcomes between peer intervention and control groups. Again, the extent to which alcohol abuse was targeted and peer education, counselling or support used was limited.

Hemrage et al. (2023) investigated psychosocial interventions to reduce alcohol use in comorbid alcohol use disorder and alcohol-related liver disease, reviewing only RCTs and focusing on drinking reduction and abstinence as intervention goals. Six databases were searched and ten RCTs were included, but only two studies focused on peer support. Nonetheless, abstinence was observed with peer support.

Turning to the studies only of school and college students, Lee et al. (2016) reviewed school-based alcohol education in 70 studies, evaluating 40 individual programs. Of these 40 programs, only three had good evidence of a positive effect – CLIMATE Schools (Australia) (an internet-based intervention), Project ALERT (USA), and All Stars (USA). Of the others, four showed some evidence of positive effect, one had no evidence of effect, 29 were inconclusive and two showed negative outcomes, such as increases in alcohol use. However, the extent to which these programs included peer education, counselling, or support was various.

The aim of Hennessy et al. (2019) was to compare seven manualized interventions for reducing problematic alcohol use among college students. They searched eight databases, including 52 RCTs, investigating the effectiveness of programs such as: The Brief Alcohol Screening Intervention for College Students (BASICS), Alcohol 101/Alcohol 101 Plus, AlcoholEdu, Check Your

Drinking, Electronic CHECKUP TO GO (e-CHUG), College Drinker's Check-up (CDCU) and Tertiary Health Research Intervention Via Email (THRIVE). These vary in length between five minutes and two hours. Six of these seven involve computer activities, while BASICS is provided through an in-person encounter. The BASICS ($n = 34$) and e-CHUG ($n = 9$) programs were the most prevalent interventions evaluated. On average, 58% of participants were male, 75% were binge drinkers, and 20% were fraternity/sorority-affiliated students. BASICS was consistently effective in reducing students' problematic alcohol use (effect size range: 0.23 – 0.36), but AlcoholEDU (effect size 0.13), e-CHUG (effect size 0.35), and THRIVE (effect size = 0.47) were also effective for some outcomes. BASICS was the most effective but was resource-intensive and might be better suited for higher-risk students.

Lavilla-Gracia et al. (2022) offered a scoping review which focused on peer-led interventions to reduce alcohol consumption for college students. Nine databases were searched for peer-led interventions that exclusively intervened in alcohol consumption, with college students as the target population. Thirteen studies were included. Only the Brief Alcohol Screening and Intervention for College Students showed a significant reduction in three of the four outcome measures: quantity and frequency of drinking, estimated peak blood alcohol concentration, and alcohol-related consequences. However, the program did not significantly decrease the number of heavy drinking episodes.

Thus, the results on these topics were mixed, with some studies showing many inconclusive results.

SINGLE STUDIES

Number of Single Studies

Several single studies were found from 1970 through 1999, but were disregarded as the cutoff for this book was 2000. From 2000, there were 13 studies from developed countries and three from developing countries.

Exemplar Single Studies Developed Context

Bobrowski et al. (2014) aimed to assess the delayed effects of two-year alcohol prevention programs implemented in Polish primary schools and homes. Both were the Polish versions of two American programs from Project Northland. The school part, led by teachers and peer leaders, comprised six sessions based on audio-taped stories told by teenagers (two boys and two girls), who described their life events, sharing their feelings and opinions. Then parent-child activities were undertaken at home. Four booklets provided information on underage drinking, alcohol advertising, peer pressure, and the consequences of alcohol consumption, containing cartoons that described the adventures of two young detectives who tried to protect children from problems. Peer leaders introduced each booklet to their classmates in school and encouraged them to participate at home. The study sample ($n = 802$) comprised 10–11-years-old pupils from eight primary schools, randomly assigned to the intervention ($n = 421$) and the control group ($n = 381$). A questionnaire was administered to students four times: at the baseline, and seven, 15, and 27 months after. At 27-month follow-up, groups were compared in terms of an increase in students who got drunk for the first time (6% in controls and 1% in the intervention group, significant). Significant changes were also found in pro-alcohol attitudes ($p = 0.043$), knowledge about the consequences of drinking ($p < 0.001$), and perceived resistance skills ($p = 0.002$).

The effect of Alcoholic Anonymous on self-management of drinking behavior in patients with alcoholic liver disease was investigated by Shen et al. (2017). Seventy-nine patients were randomly divided into controls ($n = 40$) and experimentals ($n = 39$). All patients had conventional therapy and advice on abstinence. Experimental group patients additionally had Alcoholic Anonymous intervention once a week for 12 weeks. The Michigan Alcoholism Screening Test, Motivation Assessment Questionnaire and Pennsylvania Alcohol Craving Scale were administered before and after intervention. Before intervention, there was no significant difference in all scales. After intervention, all scale scores were significantly lower in the intervention group.

Suzuki et al. (2023) noted that while inpatient alcohol withdrawal management (detoxification) was often an entry point, most patients did not successfully link to ongoing treatment. Peer recovery coaches – individuals with the lived experience of recovery who are trained to be coaches – were increasingly used and may provide a degree of continuity during this transition. An existing care coordination app (Lifeguard) was used to assist peer recovery coaches in supporting patients. Participants were contacted by the coach through the app, and after discharge received daily prompts to complete a modified version of the Brief Addiction Monitor (BAM), which enquired about alcohol use, risky and protective factors. The coach sent daily motivational texts and checked if BAM responses were concerning. All ten participants were men, averaged 50.5 years old, and were mostly White ($n = 6$) and single ($n = 8$). Eight participants successfully engaged with the coach. Following discharge, six participants continued to engage with the coach, and five responded to the BAM prompts during the follow-up. Half ($n = 5$) successfully linked with ongoing addiction treatment during follow-up. Participants who engaged with the coach post-discharge were significantly more likely to link with treatment.

Exemplar Single Studies Developing Context

Timol et al. (2016) aimed to assess the effect of an extensive, structured, time-limited, curriculum-based, peer-led educational program on first-year high school learners in public schools in the Western Cape Province of South Africa. The curriculum called 'Listen Up' addressed issues such as supporting peers and alcohol misuse in seven structured sessions, targeting adolescents in Grade 8 growing up in what are considered to be risky environments in public schools. The intervention was evaluated by ten scales sourced from published literature related to the outcome indicators of future orientation, sensation-seeking, decision-making, healthy relationships, and social support. The surveys were administered to a total of 7,709 learners across three waves of the study in 27 peer intervention schools and eight control schools. Immediately post-intervention, statistically significant differences were noted for the intervention schools when compared to their baseline levels on measures of future orientation, self-efficacy, and knowledge. Comparing baseline values with results collected between 5 and 7 months post-intervention, statistically significant results were noted for self-efficacy and knowledge.

Students in six universities in Myanmar were studied by Htet et al. (2020), exploring the prevalence of alcohol consumption and the associated risk factors. A sample of 3,456 15–24-year-old university students were selected (males 1,301 and females 2,155) and responded to a questionnaire. The prevalence of alcohol consumption in the previous 30 days was 20% (males 36%, females 11%). Alcohol consumption was significantly higher among males, truant students, smokers, and students who reported feeling of hopelessness or sadness. Peer education was seen as a way to address these issues.

Gabriel et al. (2020) explored the effect of a peer counselling intervention on the level of alcohol abuse among students in public day secondary schools in Kenya. The study targeted a population of 2,000 students who abused alcohol, from the 42 public day secondary schools in the research area. From this population, 13 peer counsellors and 600 affected students were used. Data were collected using questionnaires (e.g., the Alcohol Abuse Level Questionnaire) and interviews. The validity and reliability of these were verified prior to data collection. Where peer intervention was adequate, the subsequent rate of abstinence was 97.5% and the rate of alcohol abuse 2.5%, while where the intervention was not adequate the rate of abstinence was 40.8% and the rate of abuse 59.2%. Peer counselling as an intervention when delivered effectively had a significant positive influence on lowering the level of alcohol abuse among affected students in public day secondary schools.

SPECIFIC PROGRAM

The specific program comes from a developed country (Spain). Pueyo-Garrigues et al. (2023) conducted an RCT to assess the efficacy of a brief, peer-led alcohol intervention to reduce alcohol consumption in 50 mostly female first-year binge-drinking Spanish nursing students.

Effectiveness

Respondents were eligible if they had a binge-drinking episode in the previous month. Fifty students met this criterion and were randomly assigned to the intervention or control group. The Daily Drinking Questionnaire-Revised was used to assess the quantity of alcohol consumed on a typical weekend. Second, the Quantity/Frequency/Peak Index was used to estimate participants' maximum number of drinks consumed on the occasion of highest consumption and the number of hours they spent drinking on that occasion. Third, a closed-ended questionnaire was used to evaluate the frequency of binge-drinking episodes. Finally, the Young Adult Alcohol Consequences Questionnaire was used to evaluate issues associated with student alcohol consumption. All instruments were completed before and one month after the program. Analyses of pretest–posttest differences revealed a significant reduction in all outcome variables (alcohol consumption, binge-drinking episodes – effect size 0.69, peak Blood Alcohol Content – effect size 0.98 – and alcohol-related consequences) in the intervention group. In comparison, students in the control group exhibited a significant decrease only in the number of binge-drinking episodes. Peer counselors and participants reported high satisfaction.

Implementation

Participants randomly assigned to the intervention group received a peer-led BASICS session that consisted of a one-off 50-minute face-to-face motivational interview. A peer counselor provided participant orientation with a personalized graphical feedback sheet, with topics including the participant's: (i) drinking patterns (e.g., quantity of drinking); (ii) level of intoxication (e.g., highest blood alcohol concentration (BAC) during a typical week and heaviest drinking episode); (iii) perceived/actual drinking norms; (iv) alcohol expectancies; (v) alcohol-related consequences; (vi) individual risk factors; (vii) financial costs; (viii) alcohol calorific consumption, hours of exercise required to burn those calories; and (ix) protective behavioral strategies. Participants received a copy of their personalized feedback, a personalized BAC card, and a tips sheet (containing the most relevant alcohol information for that participant, such as supportive skills for reducing drinking-related harm).

BASICS facilitators were volunteer third- or fourth-year undergraduate nursing students who attended a pretraining course ($n = 10$). Only those who could competently conduct BASICS-based interviews and were knowledgeable about alcohol use were selected as peer counselors ($n = 4$). Their training was a workshop totaling 12 hours, administered by a mental health nurse and two counselors specializing in coaching and motivational interviews. Workshops consisted of lecture presentations, written materials, videotapes, and interactive exercises to facilitate learning of alcohol-related content and interview strategies. After training, peer counselors conducted a minimum of two videotaped practice role-playing interviews.

Peer counselors then attended two one-hour sessions where two members of the research team provided assessments of each videotaped intervention. Both tapes were coded using an alcohol-related content checklist and the Peer Proficiency Assessment. Specific instruction on the use of open-ended questions and complex reflections was provided. Peer counselors achieved proficiency in two out of three skills: the ratio of open- to closed-ended questions and the ratio of complex to simple reflexes. However, peer counselors did not achieve proficiency in the ratio of reflexes to questions. The facilitators adhered to the alcohol-related content and correctly addressed approximately 25 of the 28 total topics.

Open-ended questions elicit open-ended responses and are used to encourage students to talk without feeling defensive. Closed questions include yes/no questions and answers with a restricted range and are used to gain clarification on a specific area or gain permission to move forward in the session. Simple reflections are statements that convey understanding but offer little or no meaning (e.g., repeat, rephrase). Complex reflections are defined as statements made where substantial meaning is inferred or hypothesis testing is explored and are used to assist the student in developing discrepancy and engaging in change talk (e.g., paraphrase, double-sided reflection, reflection of feeling).

REFERENCES

Bobrowski, K. J., Pisarska, A., Staszewski, K., & Borucka, A. (2014). Effectiveness of alcohol prevention program for pre-adolescents. *Psychiatria Polska*, *48*(3), 527–539.

Gabriel, K. A., Wangila, M. J., & Risper, W. (2020). The influence of peer counseling on the level of alcohol abuse among students in public day secondary schools in imenti South sub-county. Kenya. *East African Scholars Journal of Psychology and Behavioural Sciences, 2*(3), 49–57. https://www.easpublisher. com/get-articles/1715

Hemrage, S., Brobbin, E., Deluca, P., & Drummond, C. (2023). Efficacy of psychosocial interventions to reduce alcohol use in comorbid alcohol use disorder and alcohol-related liver disease: A systematic review of randomized controlled trials. *Alcohol and Alcoholism, 58*(5), 478–484. https://doi.org/10.1093/alcalc/agad051

Hennessy, E. A., Tanner-Smith, E. E., Mavridis, D., & Grant, S. P. (2019). Comparative effectiveness of brief alcohol interventions for college students: Results from a network meta-analysis. *Prevention Science, 20*(5), 715–740. https://doi.org/ 10.1007/s11121-018-0960-z

Htet, H., Saw, Y. M., Saw, T. N., Htun, N. M. M., Lay Mon, K., & Cho, S. M., et al. (2020). Prevalence of alcohol consumption and its risk factors among university students: A cross-sectional study across six universities in Myanmar. *PLoS ONE, 15*(2), e0229329. https://doi.org/10.1371/journal.pone.0229329

Lavilla-Gracia, M., Pueyo-Garrigues, M., Pueyo-Garrigues, S., Pardavila-Belio, M. I., Canga-Armayor, A., & Esandi, N., et al. (2022). Peer-Led interventions to reduce alcohol consumption in college students: A scoping review. *Health and Social Care in the Community,* 30, e3562–e3578. https://doi.org/10.1111/ hsc.13990

Lee, N. K., Cameron, J., Battams, S., & Roche, A. (2016). What works in school-based alcohol education: A systematic review. *Health Education Journal, 75*(7), 780–798. https://doi.org/10.1177/0017896915612227

MacArthur, G. J., Harrison, S., Caldwell, D. M., Hickman, M., & Campbell, R. (2015). Peer-Led interventions to prevent tobacco, alcohol and/or drug use among young people aged 11–21 years: A systematic review and meta-analysis. *Addiction, 111*, 391–407. https://doi.org/10.1111/add.13224

Pueyo-Garrigues, S., Pardavila-Belio, M. I., Pueyo-Garrigues, M., & Canga-Armayor, N. (2023). Peer-Led alcohol intervention for college students: A pilot randomized controlled trial. *Nursing and Health Sciences,* 25, 311–322. https:// doi.org/10.1111/nhs.13023

Satinsky, E. N., Kleinman, M. B., Tralka, H. M., Jack, H. E., Myers, B., & Magidson, J. F. (2021). Peer-Delivered services for substance use in low- and middle-income countries: A systematic review. *The International Journal on Drug Policy, 95*, 103252. https://doi.org/10.1016/j.drugpo.2021.103252

Shen, J., Huang, F. F., & Wang, Z. M. (2017). The impact of alcohol abstinence mutual aid groups on self-management of drinking behavior in patients with alcoholic liver disease. *World Chinese Journal of Digestion, 25*(10), 904–908. https://doi. org/10.11569/wcjd.v25.i10.904

Suzuki, J., Loguidice, F., Prostko, S., Szpak, V., Sharma, S., & Vercollone, L., et al. (2023). Digitally assisted peer recovery coach to facilitate linkage to outpatient treatment following inpatient alcohol withdrawal treatment: Proof-of-concept pilot study. *JMIR Formative Research, 7*, e43304. https://doi.org/10.2196/43304

Timol, F., Vawda, M. Y., Bhana, A., Moolman, B., Makoae, M., & Swartz, S. (2016). Addressing adolescents' risk and protective factors related to risky behaviours: Findings from a school-based peer-education evaluation in the Western cape. *SAHARA J: Journal of Social Aspects of HIV/AIDS Research Alliance, 13*(1), 197–207. https://doi.org/10.1080/17290376.2016.1241188

Drug Use

9

DEFINITION

A drug is any substance that causes a change in physiology and/or psychology, including psychoactive changes in mood, awareness, thoughts, feelings or behavior. Some are prescribed by doctors, but many are not. They are typically self-administered (usually by swallowing, inhaling or injecting), but often have unwanted side effects. Some drugs are addictive and habit-forming, creating a compulsive need, characterized by physiological symptoms on withdrawal. Traditional "recreational" drugs include marijuana (cannabis), which is relatively mild, cocaine, which is more potent, and heroin, which is highly addictive. Others include amphetamine and methamphetamine, GHB, fentanyl, LSD, ecstasy, PCP and xylazine, with new drugs becoming available all the time. Drugs which are injected create additional dangers, such as acquiring human immunodeficiency virus (HIV)/acquired immune deficiency syndrome (AIDS) from shared needles (see Chapter 3 on HIV/AIDS). Many drugs are illegal, but trade and use are very difficult to police.

REVIEWS OF EVIDENCE

There were 11 reviews of research on drug use and abuse. An early systematic review by Cuijpers (2002) investigated school-based drug prevention programs. Three types of studies were reviewed: meta-analyses (three studies), studies examining mediating variables of interventions (six studies) and studies directly comparing prevention programs with or without specific characteristics (four studies on boosters, 12 on peer- versus adult-led programs and five on adding community interventions to school programs). Cuijpers found

---

DOI: 10.1201/9781003438366-9

that interactive delivery methods were superior, adding community interventions increased effects and the use of peer leaders was better.

A narrative review by Crawford and Bath (2013) noted that engagement between injectors and healthcare workers had been characterized by mistrust and discrimination. Peer support was one way to overcome these barriers. Peer support models had been implemented successfully, with a range of outcomes including increased treatment knowledge and uptake and improved service provision. Genuine partnerships between peers and services were common across models and led to positive transformations for both clients and services.

Reif et al. (2014) searched five databases for outcome studies of peer recovery support services 1995–2012. They found two randomized controlled trials, four quasi-experimental studies, four studies with pre-post service designs and one review. These studies met the minimum criteria for moderate level of evidence and demonstrated reduced relapse rates, increased treatment retention, improved relationships with treatment providers and social supports, and increased satisfaction with the overall treatment experience. Methodological concerns included the lack of appropriate comparison groups. Peer workers or peer helpers were people with lived experience of drug use who leverage their personal knowledge and skills to deliver harm reduction services (Marshall et al., 2015). Re specific inclusion criteria, 164 documents were selected (127 peer-reviewed and 37 gray literature references). Five categories of peer roles were identified. Current evidence provided good descriptive content but lacked systematic categorization of peer activities.

Bassuk et al. (2016) included nine studies in their review. Despite significant methodological limitations, the body of evidence suggested positive effects on participants. There had been a dramatic rise in peer support services (Tracy & Wallace, 2016), but peer support had often not been separated out as an intervention component and rigorously empirically tested. The authors searched two databases and included 10 studies from 1999. Studies showed benefits in (1) substance use, (2) treatment engagement, (3) HIV/hepatitis C virus (HCV) risk behaviors and (4) secondary substance-related behaviors such as craving and self-efficacy. Limitations were noted, especially inability to disentangle the effects of the treatment that was often included as a component of other services.

Gillespie et al. (2018) reported on opioid addiction within the city of Guelph, focusing on peer support models for harm reduction services. Several guiding principles and considerations had been established for integrating peers into harm reduction programs. Additionally, an overview of peer programs developed within North America, Europe and Australia was presented. A systematic review of peer recovery support services was offered by Eddie et al. (2019). Findings spoke tentatively to the potential of peer supports across a number of treatment settings, as evidenced by positive findings on measures, including reduced substance use and relapse rates, improved relationships with treatment providers and social supports, increased treatment retention and greater treatment satisfaction. There were however a number of null findings.

Mabuie (2020) noted that there were 13 million people who injected drugs and 1.7 million people were HIV positive. HIV transmission is higher among injectors, because of sharing equipment and risky sexual activities. Peer education drew on several theories such as information motivation behavior skill theory, the theory of reasoned action and diffusion of innovation theory. Peer educators could communicate with injectors and influence group norms. A systematic literature review searched six highly relevant research journals. Results showed peer education positively influenced the norms, attitudes and beliefs of injectors. A systematic review by Miler et al. (2020) examined peer support models within services for people impacted by homelessness and problem substance use. Six databases were searched 2000–2019, and 2,248 papers identified, of which 62 were included. The overall effectiveness and impact of peer-staffed or peer-led interventions and challenges commonly faced in these roles were investigated. Five themes relating to the challenges faced by peers were identified: vulnerability, authenticity, boundaries, stigma and lack of recognition. The findings supported involving individuals with lived experience in providing peer support to those experiencing concurrent problem substance use and homelessness.

Mercer et al. (2021) searched six databases from 2000 to 2020 and included 46 papers. Important findings included the diversity of peers' roles and the stress and trauma experienced by peers. Peers played a pivotal role in overdose prevention interventions for people who use illicit drugs but faced considerable challenges within their roles, including trauma and burnout.

SINGLE STUDIES

Number of Single Studies

There were 26 single studies, of which 19 were in developed countries and seven in developing countries.

Exemplar Single Studies Developed Context

Garfein et al. (2007) investigated whether peer education skills could reduce injection and sexual risk behaviors associated with primary HIV and HCV infection among young injection drug users. A randomized controlled trial of injectors aged 15–30 years were recruited in five US cities. A six-session, small-group, skills-building intervention in which participants were taught peer education skills (n = 431) was compared with a time-equivalent attention control (n = 423). Interviews were included for sociodemographic, psychosocial and behavioral factors during the previous 3 months; HIV and HCV antibody testing; and pre/posttest counseling. Procedures were repeated 3 and 6 months post-intervention. The intervention produced a 29% greater decline in overall injection risk 6 months post-intervention relative to the control (Odds Ratio 0.71) and a 76% decrease compared with baseline. However, overall HCV infection incidence did not differ significantly.

Injection drug users in China were studied by Shen et al. (2011). Two hundred and forty-seven drug users from a single rehabilitation center received the peer education intervention, while 420 drug users from another rehabilitation center received routine HIV/STI education and were the control. HIV/STI behavioral and knowledge domains were assessed at 3 months in rehabilitation centers after the intervention (first follow-up) and at 2–23 months in the community after release (second follow-up). Drug users who completed the intervention reported more frequent condom use with casual sex partners (60.0% vs. 12.5%, p = 0.011) and less frequent injection (56.7% vs. 26.4%, p = 0.008) at the second follow-up compared to those in the routine education group.

Hernández-Ramírez et al. (2024) sought to disentangle effects of the components of a peer-education intervention on self-reported injection risk behaviors among people who inject drugs (n = 560) in the US. They examined 226 groups/networks randomized to receive (or not) the intervention. Peer-education training consisted of two components: (1) an initial training and (2) "booster" training sessions during 6- and 12-month follow-up visits. They found that compared to control networks, among intervention networks the overall rates of injection risk behaviors were lower in both those recently exposed and those not recently exposed. However, only the boosters had statistically significant spillover effects. Thus, both intervention components reduced injection risk behaviors with evidence of spillover effects for the boosters.

Exemplar Single Studies Developing Context

Ti et al. (2013) studied HCV in Thailand with 427 participants, assessing the prevalence and factors associated with ever having been tested for HCV antibodies, for which 141 (33.0%) reported such a history. Factors positively associated with receiving a test included higher than secondary education, binge drug use, methadone treatment enrollment and having received peer-based education on HCV. The finding that injectors who received peer-based

HCV education were more likely to access HCV testing provided evidence for the value of peer-based interventions for this population.

Jarlais et al. (2016) investigated injectors in Haiphong, Vietnam, which had experienced a large HIV epidemic among injectors (68% prevalence). Interventions had reduced HIV transmission in high-income settings, but this had not been replicated in resource-limited settings. They examined strong peer support groups for identifying high-risk injectors and linking them to services. The peer support staff built and maintained trust with the participants, including recruiting, greeting and registering participants, taking electronic copies of participant fingerprints (to prevent multiple participation in the study) and conducting urinalyses. A 6-month cohort study with 250 participants followed. Peer support staff maintained contact with these participants, tracking them if they missed appointments and providing assistance in accessing methadone. Retention was high, with 86% of participants re-interviewed at 6-month follow-up. Assistance in accessing services led to half of the participants in need of methadone enrolled in methadone clinics and half of HIV-positive participants enrolled in HIV clinics by 6-month follow-up.

Pinias et al. (2022) investigated rural secondary schools in Zimbabwe, where there had been an increase in drug and substance abuse. This study examined the effectiveness of a peer counseling strategy. Twenty students and six stakeholders were purposively sampled. Document analysis and in-depth interviews revealed that both female and male students were involved in drug and substance abuse, and they influenced each other. This required empowering learners through the engagement of all stakeholders in the formulation of the peer counseling strategy. Coaching of all stakeholders on the implementation of peer counseling as an instrument to reduce students' engagement in anti-social conduct should be implemented.

SPECIFIC PROGRAM

El Mokadem et al. (2021) investigated knowledge of drugs among secondary school students in Egypt.

Effectiveness

The mean age of the participating first, second and third-grade students was 16.14 years in both experimental and control groups (males 66.7%). Peer education was implemented to improve the students' knowledge about drug abuse prevention. Results showed that there was a highly statistically significant difference between groups regarding students' knowledge about drug abuse prevention post-intervention compared to pre-intervention ($p < 0.000$). There was also a statistically significance difference between groups in the students' attitude to drug abuse prevention. There was also a high statistically significant difference between groups in student self-efficacy post-intervention. At pre-intervention, about three quarters of the study and control groups had unsatisfactory knowledge, whereas post-intervention, the majority of students in the study group (87.3%) had satisfactory knowledge compared with two-third of the students in the control group (68.7%) having unsatisfactory knowledge. More than two-thirds of the experimental students (70.3%) had negative attitudes pre-intervention, whereas post-intervention, the majority (84.3%) had positive attitudes. More than three quarters of the experimental students (78.7%) had low self-efficacy pre-intervention compared with 90.3% with high self-efficacy post-intervention. The peer education intervention was effective in enhancing knowledge, self-efficacy and attitudes of secondary school students toward drug abuse prevention.

Implementation

Peer education relies on social learning theory, which claims that modeling is an important element of the learning process. Social learning theory also asserts that some individuals function as role models of human behavior due to their ability for stimulating behavior changes in other individuals. Six secondary schools in one governorate were randomly sampled, involving 1,200 students selected from 3,200 students in the first, second and third grades. Recruited students were randomly assigned to either intervention or control group. All students were asked to nominate the most influential and compassionate students in their grade group. Those who received the most nominations were invited to become peer educators ($n = 50$).

A meeting with the peer educators explained the nature and the purpose of the study in addition to their roles as peer educators. A training week was scheduled for the peer educators. During training, peer educators were instructed on how to be sensitive, open-minded, good listeners and how to communicate their ideas and feelings in a positive and non-judgmental way, as well as how to project a positive attitude about working with their peers and how to recognize and respond to substance-related problems among friends. In addition, available sources of information and counseling services were identified so that the peer educators could guide other peers to the appropriate help. A 60-minute training session was scheduled every day for 5 days. At the end of the week, an entire day was scheduled for role playing to demonstrate how they were going to deliver the peer education intervention.

Each peer educator created a WhatsApp group to promote the program and invite students to participate. A total of 1,200 students from first, second and third grades agreed to participate in the study. Each peer educator had a group of 10–15 students, meeting after the school timetable. During the session, the peer educator explained basic information about drug abuse and ways of prevention to the students. Also, simple illustrated brochures were distributed to the students, designed by the researchers to explain the harmful effects of substance abuse, the peer pressure effect and how to say no and how to avoid engaging in any unhealthy behaviors. Each group met for two sessions over two consecutive days. The third day was planned to be an open discussion to give students a chance to ask any questions. The peer educators assured the participating students that confidentiality during the discussion would be guaranteed. The last day was designed to get the students' suggestions and feedback about the whole program.

REFERENCES

Bassuk, E. L., Hanson, J., Greene, R. N., Richard, M., & Laudet, A. (2016). Peer-Delivered recovery support services for addictions in the United States: A systematic review. *Journal of Substance Abuse Treatment*, *63*, 1–9. https://doi.org/10.1016/j.jsat.2016.01.003

Crawford, S., & Bath, N. (2013). Peer support models for people with a history of injecting drug use undertaking assessment and treatment for hepatitis C virus infection. *Clinical Infectious Diseases*, *57*(S2), S75–79. https://doi.org/10.1093/cid/cit297

Cuijpers, P. (2002). Effective ingredients of school-based drug prevention programs: A systematic review. *Addictive Behaviors*, *27*(6), 1009–1023. https://doi.org/10.1016/S0306-4603(02)00295-2

Eddie, D., Hoffman, L., Vilsaint, C., Abry, A., Bergman, B., Hoeppner, B., et al. (2019). Lived experience in new models of care for substance use disorder: A systematic review of peer recovery support services and recovery coaching. *Frontiers in Psychology*, *10*, 1052. https://doi.org/10.3389/fpsyg.2019.01052

El Mokadem, N. M., Shokr, E. A., Salama, A. H., Abo Shereda, H. M., Radwan, H. A., & Amer, H. M. (2021). Peer education intervention to promote drug abuse prevention among secondary school students. *NeuroQuantology*, *19*(5), 68–78. https://doi.org/10.14704/nq.2021.19.5.NQ21050

Garfein, R. S., Golub, E. T., Greenberg, A. E., Hagan, H., Hanson, D. L., Hudson, S. M., et al. (2007). A peer-education intervention to reduce injection risk behaviors for HIV and hepatitis c virus infection in young injection drug users. *AIDS*, *21*(14), 1923–1932. https://doi.org/10.1097/QAD.0b013e32823f9066

Gillespie, A., Lasu, B., & Sawatzky, A. (2018). *Peer support models for harm reduction services: A literature review for the Wellington Guelph Drug Strategy (WGDS)*. Guelph, ON: Community Engaged Scholarship Institute. https://atrium.lib.uoguelph.ca/xmlui/handle/10214/8902

Hernández-Ramírez, R. U., Spiegelman, D., Lok, J. J., Forastiere, L., Friedman, S. R., Latkin, C. A., et al. (2024). Overall, direct, spillover, and composite effects of components of a peer-driven intervention package on injection risk behavior among people who inject drugs in the HPTN 037 study. *AIDS and Behavior, 28*(1), 225–237. https://doi.org/10.1007/s10461-023-04213-x

Jarlais, D. D., Duong, H. T., Minh, K. P., Khuat, O. H. T., Nham, T. T. T., Arasteh, K., et al. (2016). Integrated respondent-driven sampling and peer support for persons who inject drugs in Haiphong, Vietnam: A case study with implications for interventions. *AIDS Care, 28*(10), 1312–1315. https://doi.org/10.1080/09540121.2016.1178698

Mabuie, M. A. (2020). Role of peer educators in behaviour change communication interventions for HIV prevention among people who inject drugs: Systematic review article. *Technium Social Sciences Journal, 10*, 189–200.

Marshall, Z., Dechman, M. K., Minichiello, Alcock, A. L., & Harris, G. E. (2015). Peering into the literature: A systematic review of the roles of people who inject drugs in harm reduction initiatives. *Drug and Alcohol Dependence, 151*, 1–14. http://dx.doi.org/10.1016/j.drugalcdep.2015.03.002

Mercer, F., Miler, J. A., Pauly, B., Carver, H., Hnízdilová, K., & Foster, R., et al. (2021). Peer Support and overdose prevention responses: A systematic 'state-of-the-art' review. *International Journal of Environmental Research and Public Health, 18*, 12073. https://doi.org/10.3390/ijerph182212073

Miler, J. A., Carver, H., Foster, R., & Parkes, T. (2020). Provision of peer support at the intersection of homelessness and problem substance use services: A systematic 'state of the art' review. *BMC Public Health, 20*, 641. https://doi.org/10.1186/s12889-020-8407-4.

Pinias, C., Munyaradzi, C., & Mbawuya, K. D. (2022). Exploring effectiveness of peer counselling in mitigating drug and substance abuse in Zimbabwean secondary schools: Rural learners' perspective. *E-Bangi: Journal of Social Sciences and Humanities, 19*(3), 18–32.

Reif, S., Braude, L., Lyman, D. R., Dougherty, R. H., Daniels, A. S., Ghose, S. S., et al. (2014). Peer Recovery support for individuals with substance use disorders: Assessing the evidence. *Psychiatric Services, 65*, 853–861. https://doi.org/10.1176/appi.ps.201400047

Shen, S. Y., Zhang, Z. B., Tucker, J. D., Chang, H., Zhang, G. R., & Lin, A. H. (2011). Peer-Based behavioral health program for drug users in China: A pilot study. *BMC Public Health, 11*, 693. http://www.biomedcentral.com/1471-2458/11/693

Ti, L., Kaplan, K., Hayashi, K., Suwannawong, P., Wood, E., & Kerr, T. (2013). Low rates of hepatitis c testing among people who inject drugs in Thailand: Implications for Peer-based interventions. *Journal of Public Health, 35*(4), 578–84. https://doi.org/10.1093/pubmed/fds105

Tracy, K., & Wallace, S. P. (2016). Benefits of peer support groups in the treatment of addiction. *Substance Abuse and Rehabilitation, 7*, 143–154. https://doi.org/10.2147/SAR.S81535

Smoking

10

DEFINITION

By "smoking" is meant the inhaling of tobacco smoke, which has a wide range of side effects, for example cancer, heart disease, stroke, lung diseases, diabetes, and chronic obstructive pulmonary disease (COPD), which includes emphysema and chronic bronchitis. Smoking also increases risk for tuberculosis, certain eye diseases, and problems of the immune system, including rheumatoid arthritis. Tobacco can be smoked via cigarettes, cigars, and pipes (including hookah pipes). It can also be chewed, but this has risks for the mouth rather than the lungs. Nicotine tablets are available and do not have the side effects of inhaling smoke. Smoking of other narcotic substances is dealt with under Chapter 9 Drug Abuse.

REVIEWS OF EVIDENCE

There were eight reviews of evidence on smoking, including one which focused on the co-occurring disorder of mental illness. Secker-Walker et al. (2002) reviewed community interventions for reducing smoking among adults, with a focus on reduced consumption. Of 37 studies, 23 (62%) suggested at least one favorable outcome, while 14 (38%) showed no marked difference. Increased knowledge of health risks, changes in attitudes to smoking, more attempts to quit, and better environmental and social support for quitting were not accompanied by reductions in community smoking levels. Peer supports for tobacco cessation for adults with serious mental illness were reviewed by Mackay and Dickerson (2012). The supporters also had mental health conditions. They found reports of four relevant tobacco cessation interventions. Peers were co-leaders of an educational group, individual counsellors as part of a multi-faceted tobacco treatment program, and as outreach tobacco cessation advocates. The roles of peers were promising, but more research was needed.

Ford et al. (2013) noted that smoking was disproportionately undertaken by disadvantaged communities. At that time, evidence for the effectiveness of peer or partner support interventions was equivocal. Eight studies (mostly randomized controlled trials–RCTs) were included in a systematic review. Three showed no effect, two a short-term effect, and three a medium-term effect. Improving social support for smoking cessation may be of greater importance to the disadvantaged groups. A variety of smoking prevention interventions were reviewed by Golechha (2016), who noted that smoking was more prevalent in low- or middle-income countries. Twenty-three studies were selected for inclusion. Regarding peer education, four studies were included. The Assist program was effective in the achievement of a sustained reduction in uptake of regular smoking in adolescents for two years after its delivery. Three other studies found that peer education resulted in small gains in smoking reduction.

Faseru et al. (2018) compared partners, other family members, and peers (or "buddies") as assistants in quitting by reviewing RCTs with six and/or 12-month follow-up. Fourteen studies were included. The pooled risk ratio for abstinence was 0.97 at six to nine months (i.e., slightly positive), and 1.04 at 12 months or more (i.e., slightly negative). The type of supporter did not make any difference. However, there were issues about implementation integrity. School-based interventions for adolescents in Iran were studied by Bagherinia et al. (2020). Six studies with 964 adolescents were identified for inclusion. Different methods of school education, including lectures, film presentations, group discussions, question, and answer sessions and role playing, were used. The authors assert that school-based intervention was effective, but studies largely measured self-efficacy rather than actual smoking reduction.

Huriah and Dwi (2020) also investigated school-based interventions for students aged 11–16 years with a particular focus on developing countries (Pakistan, Lebanon, Korea, Iran, Uruguay, Malaysia, and Indonesia). Smoking of cigars, smokeless tobacco, and hookah or shisha were included. There were broadly three school-based interventions: the adoption of an anti-smoking curriculum, behavior change intervention, and peer education. Only seven articles met the inclusion criteria. Three focused on peer education. There was some evidence that peer education could not only increase knowledge but also change behavior. One study, in particular, showed that the possibility of smoking was lower in the group receiving peer education interventions compared to the control group. A more rigorous review of peer support was undertaken by Yuan et al. (2023). RCTs of peer-support interventions with a smoking cessation outcome were identified, with a focus on projected abstinence at follow-up between three and nine months.

Sixteen studies were identified, which varied in abstinence effect size (risk ratio 0.61–3.07 where > 1.00 is no effect), sample size (23–2121), dose (41–207 minutes), and follow-up timepoint (<1–15 months). Across 15 trials, the risk ratio was 1.34, and effect sizes were greatest among interventions with formerly smoking peers. Peer-support interventions generally increased smoking abstinence with a modest effect sustained for all lengths of follow-up greater than six months.

SINGLE STUDIES

Number of Single Studies

There were 48 single studies of smoking. Of these, 35 (73%) were in a developed country and 13 (27%) in a developing country. Of those in a developed country, seven (20%) focused on a co-occurring condition (two cancer, two pregnancy, one HIV/AIDS/one cardiovascular risk, one homeless). Of those in a developing country, three (23%) focused on a co-occurring condition (one asthma, one mental health, one pregnancy). The references for the studies not mentioned in this chapter will be found in the Appendix.

Exemplar Single Studies Developed Context

The first two studies investigated smoking with co-occurring medical conditions. Emmons et al. (2005) explored smoking in childhood cancer survivors, who were found to smoke at rates only slightly lower than the general population. Partnership for Health was a smoking cessation intervention, a randomized control trial with follow-up at eight and 12 months that involved 796 smokers. Participants were randomly assigned to either a self-help or a peer-counselling program. The latter included up to six telephone calls from a trained childhood cancer survivor, tailored and targeted materials, and free nicotine replacement therapy. The quit rate was significantly higher in the counselling group compared with the self-help group at both eight-month and 12-month follow-up. Controlling for baseline self-efficacy and readiness to change, the intervention group was twice as likely to quit smoking. Smoking cessation rate increased in proportion to the number of counselling calls. The cost of delivering the intervention was approximately $300 per participant.

Gómez-Pardo et al. (2016) investigated a peer group intervention strategy (Fifty-Fifty) with sufferers from cardiovascular disorders. A total of 543 adults 25–50 years of age with at least one risk factor were recruited. Risk factors included hypertension (20%), overweight (82%), smoking (31%), and physical inactivity (81%). Subjects were randomized to a peer group based intervention group or a self-management control group for 12 months. Peer-elected leaders moderated monthly meetings involving role-play, brainstorming, and activities to address emotions, diet, and exercise. The primary outcome was mean change in a composite score related to blood pressure, exercise, weight, alimentation, and tobacco (Fuster-BEWAT score, 0–15). Participants' mean age was 42 years, and 71% were female. After 12 months, the intervention group score had increased and the control group score had declined (8.84 vs. 8.17, $p = 0.02$). The tobacco component particularly showed a significant difference.

Turning to studies with no co-occurring medical conditions, Orsal and Ergun (2021) conducted an RCT with 759 intervention university students in a peer education course and 1095 controls. Peer educators were trained by the researcher and her team in the Youth Friendly Center Smoking Quit Program. Students attended the treatment program voluntarily for six months. Participants in the experimental group quit smoking more than the control group ($p < 0.01$). The addiction level of the participants in the experimental group was less than that of the control group ($p < 0.01$). The intervention group gained more on the Self-Efficacy Scale, Behavior Change Process Scale, and Decision Balance Scale (all $p < 0.01$).

Apata et al. (2023) focused particularly on low-income African-American communities in the USA, who were at a greater risk than the normal population. A smoke-free policy in public housing had increased the demand for effective smoking cessation services and programs in such settings. This mixed-method pilot study explored the impact of a peer-mentoring program for smoking cessation in a public housing unit. It used a quasi-experimental design, while qualitative data were collected via focus group discussions with peer mentors and participants. Three residents of the public housing complex were trained as peer mentors. Each peer mentor recruited up to 10 smokers in the residence and provided them individual support for 12 weeks. All participants were also offered nicotine replacement therapy. A follow-up investigation was conducted three months after the intervention. Participants' smoking status was measured using self-report and verified using exhaled carbon monoxide monitoring. The intervention group had 30 current smokers and the control group had 14 individuals. Intervention mean carbon monoxide levels dropped from 26 ppm at baseline to 12 ppm at follow-up ($p < 0.01$). Participants were more likely to have non-smoking carbon monoxide levels (< 7 ppm) at follow-up (23.3%) than those who did not enroll (14.3%).

Exemplar Single Studies Developing Context

A problem with selecting studies in developing contexts is the relative weakness of such studies. Gharlipour et al. (2015) felt it important to give techniques to resist peer pressure to smoke and used the extended parallel process model of peer education. Two middle schools in Iran with all-male students were randomly selected, 120 students for the experimental group and 120 students for the control group. There was a significant difference between students in the control and experimental groups in perceived susceptibility ($p < 0.000$), perceived severity ($p < 0.000$), perceived response efficacy ($p < 0.000$), perceived self-efficacy ($p < 0.000$) and preventive behavior ($p < 0.000$). The model had a significant level of efficiency in improving preventive behavior regarding cigarette smoking among adolescents.

The Young Doctors Club was established by the Ministry of Health in Malaysia to train a group of schoolchildren as educators in assisting their peers to adopt healthy practices (Siti Nur et al., 2021). This research aimed to assess its effectiveness in a nationwide comparative cross-sectional study in instilling healthy practices among schoolchildren by identifying differences in knowledge, attitude and health practices between schools with Young Doctors Club and schools without. A questionnaire was used with 2588 year 5 (11 years old) schoolchildren from 87 primary schools nationwide, 1294 from Young Doctors Club schools and 1294 from other schools. YDC students had significantly higher overall knowledge scores and behavioral practice scores for health practices: the No Smoking component as well as hand hygiene knowledge in the particularly intervention group. Young Doctors Club schoolchildren also had significantly lower body mass index (BMI).

SPECIFIC PROGRAM

White et al. (2020) conducted an RCT to test an intervention that combined automated text messages with personalized text messages delivered by peer mentors. Thirty-eight mentors completed the online training, 36 of whom then enrolled in the study and mentored at least one participant. While the quality and timeliness of mentor communications varied markedly, there was no evidence of adverse events. Overall, 200 participants enrolled. Demographic and smoking-related characteristics of participants were balanced across study groups. Participants were predominantly female (77.5%), middle-aged (median age 45.0), non-Hispanic white (74.5%) and daily text message users (75.5%). Most participants were moderate to heavy smokers (median 15.0 cigarettes per day) and had previously attempted to quit (median three past attempts).

Efficacy of Intervention

The primary outcome of the "iQuit Project" was biochemically verified seven-day abstinence at three months, which was 7.9% in the intervention group and 3.0% in the control group. Adjusting for baseline characteristics, abstinence was 6.5 percentage points higher in the mentor group than the control group ($p = 0.03$), a 260% increase over the 2.5% abstinence in the control group. Self-reported seven-day abstinence at three months was 23.8% in the intervention group and 13.1% in the control group. Adjusting for baseline characteristics, self-reported abstinence was 12.7 percentage points higher in the intervention group than the control group ($p = 0.03$), a 99% increase over the 12.8% abstinence in the control group. Intervention participants also experienced fewer cravings and better mood than the control group.

Implementation

Participants were recruited primarily from paid advertisements placed on Google and Facebook. Recruitment notices were also disseminated through various American Cancer Society (ACS) webpages, the SmokefreeTXT sign-up webpage and Facebook webpages dedicated to smoking cessation. All advertisements directed participants to the study website, which included study details and a screening survey.

Inclusion criteria were age ≥ 18 years, living in the United States, having smoked ≥ 100 cigarettes in their lifetime, being a current cigarette smoker, wanting to quit within 30 days, not having used nicotine replacement therapy or electronic nicotine delivery systems within the past 30 days, and agreeing to complete a salivary cotinine test at three-month follow-up. Eligible participants gave informed consent and completed a web-based baseline questionnaire.

Peer mentors were recruited from multiple sources: solicitation of facilitators of the ACS Freshstart® group-based cessation support program, online notices on ACS webpages and posts to online smoking cessation forums. Eligibility criteria for mentors were age ≥ 18 years, living in the US, having quit smoking > 1 year, willingness to mentor smokers through texting, completing the online training program and creating a personal profile.

The training for mentors included six narrated modules with an accompanying slide deck that took roughly two hours to complete, with a quiz at the end of each module. The modules covered study details, information about smoking and smoking cessation, guidance rooted in motivational interviewing techniques regarding how to advise mentees and a tutorial about the study's web-based text-messaging platform. Study investigators verified that mentors had completed each quiz (i.e., each training module) before enrolling them in the study.

Participants were randomly allocated to receive cessation assistance through an automated texting program plus peer mentoring ($n = 101$) or an automated texting program alone ($n = 99$). Mentor assignment was also random. Participants were informed of their group and mentor assignment at the end of the baseline questionnaire.

Text messages were based on SmokefreeTXT (SFTXT), a nationwide text-messaging service provided by the National Cancer Institute (NCI). SFTXT provides emotional and educational support concordant with the US clinical practice guidelines for smoking cessation and uses 41 different behavior change techniques, including goal setting, problem solving, self-monitoring, feedback and social support. SFTXT delivers one to five automated messages per day for up to two weeks prior to a user-selected quit date and six weeks post-quit date. A key feature of SFTXT, also incorporated in texts sent to both study groups, is that users are periodically sent messages to assess their smoking, mood and craving status. Responses to status assessment messages prompt an automatic reply. Individuals can also request additional messages. For the intervention, the SFTXT message library was imported into Wellpass, a secure online portal designed for patient–clinician interactions. Wellpass allows for scheduled messages and automated dynamic responses. Participants also had the option to receive their messages through Wellpass' instant messaging smartphone app.

During baseline, participants selected a quit date within the next 5–15 days, with a default option of 15 days to maximize preparation time. A welcome text message was sent upon enrolment and the SFTXT-based script began on the following day. Participants in the control group received an identical set of text messages to SFTXT but no other intervention component. Participants in the intervention group received a modified version of the SFTXT messages and assignment to a peer mentor. At start-up, intervention participants were automatically redirected to a webpage with their assigned mentor's profile. A link to the profile webpage was also sent to participants by email and within the welcome text message.

Subsequently, intervention participants received a combination of automated and personalized text messages, identical to SFTXT's, except that they included five enhancements. First, the messages were more conversational in tone. Second, one automated message each day was to be a "conversation starter" that prompted users to reply. For example, one message asks users, "What are your top 3 smoking triggers?" All participant replies triggered an email push notification to the mentor. Prior to the trial, mentors received a message library, along with examples of follow-up prompts and probes that could be employed with each conversation starter. Third, information was solicited from mentors regarding their own experiences with quitting, and the content embedded into selected messages. For example, one message read: "Think of healthy ways to deal with stress & boredom instead of smoking. For instance, go to the gym, take a jog, or walk the dog." However, the mentor's own stress relief techniques could be inserted in the second sentence. This personalized content was designed to build a social bond between mentor and participant and to make the participant more comfortable with sharing personal experiences. Fourth, mentors could remove or edit automated messages to tailor them to each participant. Fifth, mentors could send spontaneous (unscripted) messages at any time.

Mentors received an email notification when assigned a new participant, including a brief mentee profile with demographic data (first name, gender, age, race, time zone, whether a daily smoker, average cigarettes per day, years smoking, reason for smoking, reason for wanting to quit, quit methods of potential interest and quit date). If a mentor did not accept an assigned participant, study personnel sent a reminder after one day and assigned the participant to a new mentor after two days. Back-up mentors were kept in reserve for this purpose. Study personnel monitored chat logs daily and contacted mentors by email if they went more than a day without responding to participant questions.

The intervention lasted 42 days. Smoking status assessment messages continued at day 60 and day 90. On day 91, participants received an email message with a link to the follow-up questionnaire. For those who had not responded yet, there was follow-up in a staggered fashion with three emails, two text messages and two phone calls. Self-reported abstainers at follow-up were mailed a salivary cotinine test kit. Participants received a $25 gift card for completing the follow-up and an additional $25 for sending by email a photograph of their salivary test results. Mentors received $50 for completing the training, $150 for mentoring ($200 for accepting four mentees) and entry into a $1000 draw.

REFERENCES

Apata, J., Goldman, E., Taraji, H., Samagbeyi, O., Assari, S., & Sheikhattari, P. (2023). Peer Mentoring for smoking cessation in public housing: A mixed-methods study. *Frontiers in Public Health, 10,* 1052313. https://doi.org/10.3389/fpubh.2022.1052313

Bagherinia, M., Simbar, M., Yazdani, F., Safajou, F., & Mohamadkhani Shahri, L. (2020). Effectiveness of school-based educational interventions in preventing smoking in Iranian adolescents: A systematic review. *International Journal of Pediatrics, 8*(11), 12421–430. https://doi.org/10.22038/ijp.2020.46355.3773

Emmons, K. M., Puleo, E., Park, E., Gritz, E. R., Butterfield, R. M., Weeks, J. C., Mertens, A., & Li, F. P. (2005). Peer-Delivered smoking counseling for childhood cancer survivors increases rate of cessation: The partnership for health study. *Journal of Clinical Oncology, 23*(27), 6516–6523. https://doi.org/10.1200/JCO.2005.07.048

Faseru, B., Richter, K. P., Scheuermann, T. S., & Park, E. W. (2018). Enhancing partner support to improve smoking cessation. Cochrane Tobacco Addiction Group, ed. *Cochrane Database of Systematic Reviews*, 8. Art. No.: CD002928. https://doi.org/10.1002/14651858.CD002928.pub4

Ford, P., Clifford, A., Gussy, K., & Gartner, C. (2013). A systematic review of peer-support programs for smoking cessation in disadvantaged groups. *International Journal of Environmental Research and Public Health*, *10*, 5507–5522. https://doi.org/10.3390/ijerph10115507

Gharlipour, Z., Hazavehei, S. M., Moeini, B., Nazari, M., Beigi, A. M., & Tavassoli, E., et al. (2015). The effect of a preventive educational program in cigarette smoking: Extended parallel process model. *Journal of Education and Health Promotion*, *4*(4). https://doi.org/10.4103/2277-9531.151875

Golechha, M. (2016). Health promotion methods for smoking prevention and cessation: A comprehensive review of effectiveness and the way forward. *International Journal of Preventive Medicine*, *7*(1), 7. https://doi.org/10.4103/2008-7802.173797

Gómez-Pardo, E., Fernández-Alvira, J. M., Vilanova, M., Haro, D., Martínez, R., & Carvajal, I., et al. (2016). A comprehensive lifestyle peer group-based intervention on cardiovascular risk factors: The randomized controlled fifty-fifty program. *Journal of the American College of Cardiology*, *67*(5), 476–485. https://doi.org/10.1016/j.jacc.2015.10.033

Huriah, T., & Dwi, L. V. (2020). School-based smoking prevention in adolescents in developing countries: A literature review. *Macedonian Journal of Medical Science*, *8*(F), 84–89. https://oamjms.eu/index.php/mjms/article/view/4336

Mackay, C. E., & Dickerson, F. (2012). Peer Supports for tobacco cessation for adults with serious mental illness: A review of the literature. *Journal of Dual Diagnosis*, *8*(2), 104–112. https://doi.org/10.1080/15504263.2012.670847

Orsal, O., & Ergun, A. (2021). The effect of peer education on decision-making, smoking-promoting factors, self-efficacy, addiction, and behavior change in the process of quitting smoking of young people. *Risk Management and Healthcare Policy*, *14*, 925–945. https://doi.org/10.2147/RMHP.S280393

Siti Nur, F., Shubash, S., Noorlaile, Normawati, Zaman, K., Bakar, A., Suraiya, & Manimaran, K. (2021). Evaluating the effectiveness of peer education program on health knowledge, attitudes and practices. *Global Journal of Health Science*, *13*(1), 74. https://doi.org/10.5539/gjhs.v13n1p74

Secker-Walker, R. H., Gnich, W., Platt, S., & Lancaster, T. (2002). Community interventions for reducing smoking among adults. *Cochrane Database of Systematic Reviews*, 2. Art. No.: CD001745. https://doi.org/10.1002/14651858.CD001745

White, J. S., Toussaert, S., Thrul, J., Bontemps-Jones, J., Abroms, L., & Westmaas, J. L. (2020). Peer Mentoring and automated text messages for smoking cessation: A randomized pilot. *Nicotine & Tobacco Research*, *22*(3), 371–380. https://doi.org/10.1093/ntr/ntz047

Yuan, P., Westmaas, J. L., Thrul, J., Toussaert, S., Hilton, J. F., & White, J. S. (2023). Effectiveness of peer-support interventions for smoking cessation: A systematic review and meta-analysis. *Nicotine and Tobacco Research*, *25*, 1515–1524. https://doi.org/10.1093/ntr/ntad059

Obesity and Physical Activity

11

DEFINITION

Obesity is defined as abnormal or excessive fat accumulation that presents a risk to health. A body mass index (BMI) over 25 is considered overweight and over 30 is considered obese. Rates of overweight and obesity continue to grow in adults and children in the world. From 1990 to 2022, the percentage of children and adolescents aged 5–19 years living with obesity increased four-fold from 2% to 8% globally, while the percentage of adults 18 years of age and older living with obesity more than doubled from 7% to 16%. Overweight and obesity are major risk factors for a number of chronic diseases, including cardiovascular diseases such as heart disease and stroke, which are the leading causes of death worldwide. Being overweight can also lead to diabetes and its associated conditions, including blindness, limb amputations and the need for dialysis. Rates of diabetes have quadrupled since around the world since 1980. Carrying excess weight can lead to musculoskeletal disorders including osteoarthritis. Obesity is also associated with some cancers.

As global diets have changed in recent decades, there has been an increase in the consumption of energy-dense foods high in fat and sugar. There has also been a decrease in physical activity due to the changing nature of many types of work and easier access to transportation. Reducing obesity involves lowering or changing food intake and increasing physical activity. Lowering or changing food intake is dealt with in Chapter 12 on Breastfeeding and Nutrition. Interventions to increase physical activity have become more necessary and more widespread in recent years, whether to prevent or reduce obesity. Physical activity can be defined as any bodily movement produced by skeletal muscles that increases power/energy spending.

DOI: 10.1201/9781003438366-11

Studies on reducing obesity and on enhancing physical activity are dealt with in separate sub-sections, but they are categorized in accordance with the search term which first highlighted their existence and the division between them is sometimes rather arbitrary, so readers should expect some cross-over.

REVIEWS OF EVIDENCE

There were seven reviews on obesity and ten reviews on physical activity. It is interesting that there are more reviews on preventive than corrective concerns, but the majority of studies on physical activity come from developed countries, which is not true of obesity.

Obesity

Nickols-Richardson et al. (2014) conducted a systematic review from 1977 to 2013 on nutrition- and obesity-related outcomes in youth. They included 15 studies, reporting various methods of selecting, training and assigning responsibilities to peer educators. There were some studies showing peer education improved attitudes, perceptions and self-efficacy for healthy eating. A critical review of results from youth peer-led lifestyle modification and weight management programs was offered by Vangeepuram et al. (2020). However, they only searched one database from 2002 to 2015, identifying 29 interventions for children from kindergarten to 12th grade. Youth peer-led interventions could result in positive changes in behavior, diet, physical activity, body measures and other clinical outcomes. It was recommended that peer leaders receive extensive training and regular supervision.

Lim et al. (2021) aimed to meta-analyze the efficacy of peer interventions on body weight, energy intake and physical activity in adults, searching 14 databases and including 65 articles. Peer interventions resulted in significant reduction in weight (28 studies), BMI (25 studies), waist circumference (12 studies) and a significant increase in physical activity (41 studies), but with no significant effect on energy intake. In the same year, Chen et al. (2021) conducted a meta-analysis on weight, BMI, waist circumference, blood pressure, quality of life, social support and depressive symptoms. They searched three databases to 2020 and included 14 randomized controlled trials (RCTs).

A significant improvement in weight was found in individuals who received peer support compared to usual care ($p = 0.02$). Peer support was also associated with significant decrease in BMI ($p = 0.04$). However, there was no statistically significant improvement in the levels of waist circumference, systolic blood pressure, diastolic blood pressure, quality of life, social support and depressive symptoms.

Martin-Vicario and Gómez-Puertas (2022) reviewed two databases from 2011 to 2021, selecting 21 studies and focusing on the effects of social support for members of obesity online health communities. Social support improved weight loss, behavioral change and community participation. This study pointed to both a direct and indirect relationship between social support in online health communities and actual weight loss. A meta-analysis of peer-led interventions on child and adolescent obesity was reviewed by Nguyen et al. (2022). They included 14 studies with a minimum duration of four weeks and reported on BMI, all from high-income countries. The meta-analysis showed effectiveness ($p = 0.01$). There were significantly greater effects from interventions focusing on physical activity alone or with longer duration of implementation.

One outlier review focused on obesity in people with serious mental illness (Stubbs et al., 2016), focused on peer intervention on physical health, lifestyle factors and appointment attendance. A systematic search to 2016 resulted in seven studies being included, including three RCTs. There was considerable heterogeneity in the type of peer support and the role of the peer support workers. Three studies found insignificant reductions in weight. Evidence from another three studies on lifestyle changes was equivocal, only one study demonstrating improved self-reported physical activity and diet. Evidence regarding appointment attendance was also unclear across four studies.

Physical Activity

Ginis et al. (2013) included ten published studies. In all studies reporting within-group analyses, peer-delivered interventions led to increases in physical activity. Peer-delivered interventions were just as effective as professionally delivered interventions and more effective than control conditions for increasing physical activity. Three studies yielded evidence that peers may enhance self-efficacy and self-determination. School-based peer interventions were systematically reviewed by Jenkinson et al. (2014). Only four RCTs were identified, and only two other studies had control groups. Nine of the 19 studies reported significant findings.

Tutor training varied considerably; 13 of the 19 studies provided some training. Mendonca et al. (2014) searched eight databases to 2011 and 75 studies were included. Social support was consistently associated with the physical activity level of adolescents in cross-sectional and longitudinal studies. Those who received more support showed higher levels of physical activity.

Three information databases in Iran were searched by Abdi et al. (2015) from 2003 to 2013; 20 studies were included. Almost all studies used self-reporting instruments. None of the studies assessed the effectiveness of educational methods. Behavior maintenance was not addressed in 75% of the studies. Best et al. (2016) systematically reviewed and meta-analyzed outcomes, searching six databases for RCTs and including 21 studies. Statistically significant improvements in physical activity were reported by 14 studies. A meta-analysis of 17 studies showed a statistically significant pooled effect size (0.4, $p < 0.001$) immediately post-intervention. A large effect was evident in the four studies that included follow-up measures (1.5, $p = 0.03$).

A focus on older people came from Burton et al. (2017). The systematic review and meta-analysis covered 1976–2016 from six databases including 18 studies. Average participant age was 66.5 years and 67% were female. Interventions included resistance, flexibility and cardiovascular training. Hulteen et al. (2019) searched eight databases for five years from 2018, including 15 studies. Peer-delivered interventions appeared to represent an efficacious means of promoting physical activity among diverse populations across the lifespan, and in different settings. A scoping review by Tweed et al. (2020) searched four databases 2007–2019, including 13 studies. Nine studies found a significant increase in perceived social support, seven studies reported increased mental wellbeing and five studies reported increased physical activity levels. Gains also included exercise-related psychosocial benefits, knowledge relating to selfcare and improved social connections.

Christensen et al. (2020) focused on youth, conducting a scoping review including 43 studies. Youth peer leadership initiatives could increase physical activity for youth and children. Similarly, McHale et al. (2022) focused on adolescents, searching three databases for studies reporting at least one outcome in 12- to 19-year-olds and including 18 studies. Half ($n = 9$) reported improved outcomes in the school setting. The most prominent behavioral change techniques were social support, information about health consequences and demonstration of the behavior. Both cross-age and same-age interventions seemed effective. Gender-specific interventions showed great promise.

SINGLE STUDIES

Number of Single Studies

There were 39 single studies on obesity and 46 on physical activity. In obesity, 14 out of 39 studies (36%) were from developing countries or focused on disadvantaged communities (this relatively high proportion reflecting the global concern with this issue), while 25 were from developed countries. In physical activity, six out of 46 studies (13%) were from developing countries or focused on disadvantaged communities (this relatively low proportion reflecting a lesser preoccupation with preventive studies in developing countries), while 40 were from developed countries.

Exemplar Single Studies Developed Context

Mothers in Motion (MIM), a community-based intervention program, was designed by Chang et al. (2019) to help young, low-income women with overweight or obesity prevent further weight gain by promoting stress management, healthy eating and physical activity. This study reports MIM's effect on self-efficacy to cope with stress, emotional coping response, social support for stress management, stress, depressive symptoms and positive and negative affect. Participants ($n = 612$) were recruited in Michigan, USA, and randomly assigned to an intervention group (410 participants) or a comparison group (202 participants). During the 16-week intervention, intervention participants watched ten video lessons at home and joined ten peer support group teleconferences. Surveys with established validity and reliability were used to measure self-efficacy to cope with stress, emotional coping response and social support for stress management at the end of the 16-week intervention and at three-month follow-up. At post-test, the intervention group reported significantly higher self-efficacy to cope with stress (effect size $d = 0.53$), better emotional coping response ($d = 0.38$), less stress ($d = 0.34$), fewer depressive symptoms ($d = -0.27$) and more positive affect ($d = 0.31$) than the comparison group. However, there were no significant differences in social support for stress management or negative affect. At follow-up, the intervention group still reported significantly higher self-efficacy to cope with stress ($d = 0.32$) and better emotional coping response ($d = 0.34$) than the comparison group but did not report significantly higher social support for stress management, stress, depressive symptoms, or positive and negative affect.

Huitink et al. (2021) noted that supermarkets located near schools influenced adolescents' food consumption. Their study aimed to (1) measure dietary behaviors during school hours, (2) to investigate the effect of a nutrition peer-education intervention in supermarkets within walking distance to secondary schools on nutritional knowledge and attitudes toward healthy eating and (3) to assess how the intervention was appraised by adolescents with a lower education level. The participants were adolescents aged 12–14 years from four secondary schools (n = 432). Cross-sectional analyses were performed to establish dietary behaviors (pretest). A quasi-experimental pre–post design with a comparison school was used. Intervention schools received the intervention in a supermarket near their school. Most of the adolescents who purchased foods from retail food outlets near the school (71%) did so from supermarkets (89%). The nutritional knowledge scores (p = 0.003) as well as the attitudes toward healthy eating (p = 0.009) of adolescents from the intervention schools were statistically significantly higher after the intervention, relative to the comparison school.

Whether tailored support from older peer volunteers could improve initiation and long-term maintenance of physical activity behavior for older adults was examined by Buman et al. (2021). Participants were randomized to two 16-week, group-based programs: (1) peer-delivered, theory-based support for physical activity behavior change; or (2) an intervention typically available in community settings (basic education, gym membership and pedometer for self-monitoring), attention-matched with health education. Moderate-to-vigorous physical activity (MVPA) was assessed via daily self-report logs at baseline, at the end of the intervention (16 weeks) and at follow-up (18 months), with accelerometry validation in a random subsample. Seven peer volunteers and 81 sedentary adults were recruited. Retention at the end of the trial was 85% and at follow-up at 18 months 61%. At 16 weeks, both groups had similar significant improvements in MVPA. At 18 months, the group supplemented with peer support had significantly more MVPA.

Exemplar Single Studies Developing Context

Jeihooni et al. (2015) aimed to determine the effect of peer education on nutrition and physical activity in 200 obese and overweight female high school students, randomly assigned to control and experimental groups. Peer intervention occurred in ten educational sessions of 50–55 minutes. The physical activity and nutrition performances questionnaire was completed before and three months after. Before educational intervention, there were no significant differences between experimental and control groups in knowledge, attitude, self-efficacy, enabling factors, reinforcing factors, physical and nutrition performances. However, three months after the intervention, the experimental group showed significant enhancement in all of these compared to the control group. Pre-intervention, there were no significant differences in weight and BMI between the experimental and control groups, but post-intervention, there were significant differences in the experimental group, while the control group had no changes.

Gunawardena et al. (2016) developed a program that enabled school children to act as change agents in promoting healthy lifestyles in their mothers, measured by weight, physical activity and dietary habit. A 12-month cluster randomized trial was conducted, with school as a cluster. Participants were mothers of grade 8 students (aged around 13 years) in 20 schools in Sri Lanka. Students were trained to acquire the ability to assess non-communicable disease risk factors in their homes and take action to address them. Body weight, step count and lifestyle of the mothers were assessed at baseline and post-intervention. Of 308 study participants, 261 completed the final assessment at 12 months. There was a significantly greater decrease of weight and increase of physical activity in the intervention group. The intervention group had 3.25 times higher odds of engaging in adequate physical activity than the control group and showed a greater number of steps than the latter. The effect sizes were 2.49 for weight and 0.99 for BMI. The intervention group showed a greater reduction of household purchase of biscuits and ice cream.

Older people with type 2 diabetes were studied by Sazlina et al. (2015), who compared personalized feedback alone or with peer support. A three-arm randomized controlled trial was conducted in Malaysia. Sixty-nine sedentary Malays aged 60 years and older who received usual care were randomized to feedback or feedback + support interventions or served as controls for 12 weeks, with follow-ups at weeks 24 and 36. Intervention groups performed unsupervised walking activity and received written feedback on physical activity. The feedback + peer support group also received group and telephone contacts from trained peer mentors. The primary outcome was pedometer steps. Secondary outcomes were self-reported physical activity, cardiovascular risk factors, cardiorespiratory fitness, balance, quality of life and psychosocial wellbeing. Fifty-two participants (75%) completed the study. The feedback + peer support group showed greater daily pedometer readings than the feedback and control groups ($p = 0.001$). This group also had greater improvement in weekly duration ($p < 0.001$) and frequency ($p < 0.001$) of moderate intensity physical activity, scores on the Physical Activity Scale for Elderly ($p = 0.003$), six-minute walk test ($p < 0.001$) and social support from friends ($p = 0.032$).

SPECIFIC PROGRAM

The specific program was in obesity and other areas and was drawn from a developed country.

Effectiveness

A cluster RCT was conducted by Diao et al. (2020), involving 1,564 subjects who were divided into an intervention group ($n = 714$) and a control group ($n = 850$). The intervention group received a full year of peer education. Their quality of life (QoL) was assessed using the Adolescent Quality of Life Scale and a self-designed basic situation questionnaire. After the intervention, significant increases were found in the psychological effects ($p = 0.013$) and in total QoL ($p = 0.016$) in the intervention group relative to the control group. However, no significant changes were observed for the social QoL of both groups and the total QoL of the control group ($p > 0.05$).

Implementation

The cluster RCT involved four schools (two primary schools, two junior middle schools) and were randomly divided into intervention and control groups. The study began in grades 4–5 (primary) and grades 7–8 (junior middle). The average age of the participants was 12.5 years. A total of 1,789 students were eligible to participate, but nine were excluded on the grounds of mental retardation. After one year of peer education, a follow-up was carried out on the same subjects. The baseline survey was done with 787 intervention students and 993 control students, who completed a 40-minute QoL questionnaire. The reliability and validity of the QoL scale was assessed in other primary and junior middle schools, resulting in alpha coefficients of the physical, social, psychological and pubertal dimensions and whole scale at 0.81, 0.77, 0.85, 0.64 and 0.89, respectively. The retest reliability values were 0.76, 0.78, 0.82, 0.72 and 0.88, respectively. The intervention was then initiated and completed three months later. The final assessment was conducted nine months later.

Following discussions with class teachers, the researchers selected four excellent, prestigious and well-communicated students (two boys and two girls) who were class committee members and actively participated in extra-curricular activities, who were asked to act as peer educators. Adolescent health education training for the peer educators was conducted and its effectiveness evaluated. The results showed the correct knowledge and the attitudes of the peer educators significantly improved. Secondly, the forms of peer education included knowledge contests, group discussions, role-playing and self-made poster exhibitions based on adolescent health education (knowledge quiz software was provided, as were group discussion cases and analysis results, role-playing scripts and related pubertal health education slides). Peer educators utilized the class meeting or spare time to perform related activities among their peers. After each activity, the peer educators recorded key information, including the number of participants, the content of the discussions and whether the peers showed relevant knowledge acquisition. Each class was required to have at least two activities per month. Thirdly, secondary peer educator training was performed to consolidate relevant knowledge and included knowledge regarding mental resilience, teaching and how to cope with stress or negative events. Finally, supervision of the peer educators was carried out twice per semester to assess progress and collect evidence of activities, including activity records, adolescent posters and activity photos. The average number of activities per class was 20, ranging from 8 to 50. Each class developed 5.5 posters on average, with minimum values of four posters and maximum values of eight posters per class.

Physiological knowledge, psychological health education and health lifestyles were the three areas targeted. Physiological health education included growth spurts, the development of secondary sexual characteristics, acne treatment, "how to treat breast development, menstruation and dysmenorrhea for girls", "how to deal with beard growth and spermatorrhea for boys" and cleaning of the private parts. Psychological health education involved characteristics of adolescent psychological development and "how to deal with common psychological problems such tension, anxiety and conflicts with parents, teachers and companions"; health lifestyle included a balanced diet, reasonable exercise and keeping good sleeping patterns (see online resource: https://doi.org/10.1007/s11136-019-02309-3).

REFERENCES

Abdi, J., Eftekhar, H. E., Estebsari, F., & Sadeghi, R. (2015). Theory-based interventions in physical activity: A systematic review of literature in Iran. *Global Journal of Health Science, 7*(3), 215–229. https://doi.org/10.5539/gjhs.v7n3p215

Best, K. L., Miller, W. C., Eng, J. J., & Routhier, F. (2016). Systematic review and meta-analysis of peer-led self-management programs for increasing physical activity. *International Journal of Behavioral Medicine, 23*, 527–538. https://doi.org/10.1007/s12529-016-9540-4.

Buman, M. P., Giacobbi, P. R., Dzierzewski, J. M., Morgan, A. A., McCrae, C. S., Roberts, B. L., et al. (2011). Peer volunteers improve long-term maintenance of physical activity with older adults: A randomized controlled trial. *Journal of Physical Activity and Health*, *8*(Suppl 2), S257–S266. https://doi.org/10.1123/jpah.8.s2.s257

Burton, E., Farrier, K., Hill, K., Codde, J., Airey, P., & Hill, A. (2017). Effectiveness of peers in delivering programs or motivating older people to increase their participation in physical activity: Systematic review and meta-analysis. *Journal of Sports Sciences*, *36*(6), 666–678. https://doi.org/10.1080/02640414.2017.1329549

Chang, M. W., Nitzke, S., & Brown, R. (2019). Mothers in motion: Intervention effect on psychosocial health in young, low-income women with overweight or obesity. *BMC Public Health*, *19*, 56. https://doi.org/10.1186/s12889-019-6404-2.

Chen, Y., Li, Z., Yang, Q., Yang, S., Dou, C., & Zhang, T., et al. (2021). The effect of peer support on individuals with overweight and obesity: A meta-analysis. *Iranian Journal of Public Health, 50*(12), 2439–2450. https://doi.org/10.18502/ijph.v50i12.7926

Christensen, J. H., Elsborg, P., Melby, P. S., Nielsen, G., & Bentsen, P. (2020). A scoping review of peer-led physical activity interventions involving young people: Theoretical approaches, intervention rationales, and effects. *Youth & Society*, *53*(5), 811–840. https://doi.org/10.1177/0044118X20901735

Diao, H., Pu, Y., Yang, L. J., Ting Li, T., Jin, F., & Wang, H. (2020). The impacts of peer education based on adolescent health education on the quality of life in adolescents: A randomized controlled trial. *Quality of Life Research*, *29*, 153–161. https://doi.org/10.1007/s11136-019-02309-3

Ginis, K. A. M., Nigg, C. R., & Smith, A. L. (2013). Peer-delivered physical activity interventions: An overlooked opportunity for physical activity promotion. *TBM*, *3*, 434–443. https://doi.org/10.1007/s13142-013-0215-2

Gunawardena, N., Kurotani, K., Indrawansa, S., Nonaka, D., Mizoue, T., & Samarasinghe, D. (2016). School-based intervention to enable school children to act as change agents on weight, physical activity and diet of their mothers: A cluster randomized controlled trial. *International Journal of Behavioral Nutrition and Physical Activity*, *13*, 45. https://doi.org/10.1186/s12966-016-0369-7

Huitink, M., Poelman, M. P., Seidell, J. C., & Dijkstra, S. C. (2021). The healthy supermarket coach: Effects of a nutrition peer-education intervention in Dutch supermarkets involving adolescents with a lower education level. *Health Education & Behavior*, *48*(2), 150–159. https://doi.org/10.1177/1090198120957953

Hulteen, R. H., Waldhauser, K. J., & Beauchamp, M. R. (2019). Promoting health-enhancing physical activity: A state-of-the-art review of peer-delivered interventions. *Current Obesity Reports*, *8*, 341–353. https://doi.org/10.1007/s13679-019-00366-w

Jeihooni, A. K., Heidari, M. S., Harsini, P. A., & Azizinia, S. (2019). Application of PRECEDE model in education of nutrition and physical activities in obesity and overweight female high school students. *Obesity Medicine*, *14*, 100092. https://doi.org/10.1016/j.obmed.2019.100092

Jenkinson, K. A., Naughton, G., & Benson, A. C. (2014). Peer-Assisted learning in school physical education, sport and physical activity programmes: A systematic review. *Physical Education and Sport Pedagogy, 19*(3), 253–277. https://doi.org/10.1080/17408989.2012.754004

Lim, S., Lee, W. K., Tan, A., Chen, M. L., Tay, C. T., Sood, S., et al. (2021). Peer-Supported lifestyle interventions on body weight, energy intake, and physical activity in adults: A systematic review and meta-analysis. *Obesity Reviews, 22*, e13328. https://doi.org/10.1111/obr.13328

Martin-Vicario, L., & Gómez-Puertas, L. (2022). The role of social support in obesity online health communities: A literature review. *Review of Communication Research, 10*, 146–171.

McHale, F., Ng, K., Taylor, S., Bengoechea, E., Norton, C., O'Shea, D., et al. (2022). A systematic literature review of peer-led strategies for promoting physical activity levels of adolescents. *Health Education & Behavior, 49*(1), 41–53.

Mendonca, G., Cheng, L. A., Me´lo, E. N., & de Farias, J. C. (2014). Physical activity and social support in adolescents: A systematic review. *Health Education Research, 29*(5), 822–839. https://doi.org/10.1093/her/cyu017

Nguyen, N. M., Dibley, M. J., Tang, H. K., & Alam, A. (2022). Effectiveness of peer-led programs for overweight and obesity in children: Systematic review and meta-analysis. *International Journal of Obesity, 46*(12), 2070–2087. https://doi.org/10.1038/s41366-022-01219-8

Nickols-Richardson, S. M., Nelson, S. A., & Corbin, M. A. (2014). Peer Nutrition education in childhood and adolescence: Evidence-based guidance for impactful programs. *Journal of Nutrition Education and Behavior, 46*(4), S196. https://doi.org/10.1016/j.jneb.2014.04.211

Sazlina, S. G., Browning, C. J., & Yasin, S. (2015). Effectiveness of personalized feedback alone or combined with peer support to improve physical activity in sedentary older malays with type 2 diabetes: A randomized controlled trial. *Frontiers in Public Health, 3*, 178. https://doi.org/10.3389/fpubh.2015.00178

Stubbs, B., Williams, J., Shannon, J., Gaughran, F., & Craig, T. (2016). Peer Support interventions seeking to improve physical health and lifestyle behaviours among people with serious mental illness: A systematic review. *International Journal of Mental Health Nursing, 25*(6), 484–495. https://doi.org/10.1111/inm.12256

Tweed, L. M., Rogers, E. N., & Kinnafick, F. E. (2020). Literature on peer-based community physical activity programmes for mental health service users: A scoping review. *Health Psychology Review, 5*(2), 287–313. https://doi.org/10.1080/17437199.2020.1715812

Vangeepuram, N., Angeles, J., Lopez-Belin, P., Arniella, G., & Horowitz, C. R. (2020). Youth peer led lifestyle modification interventions: A narrative literature review. *Evaluation and Program Planning, 83*, 101871. https://doi.org/10.1016/j.evalprogplan.2020.101871

Breastfeeding and Nutrition

12

DEFINITION

Breastfeeding

Breastfeeding is the process where milk from the mother's breasts is fed to a child. Breast milk may be immediately from the breast or may be pumped and fed to the infant later. The World Health Organization recommends that breastfeeding begins within the first hour of a baby's birth. Breast milk contains vitamins and minerals, offers protection from certain infections, helps improve the baby's long-term health and reduces the risk of sudden infant death syndrome, childhood diabetes and leukemia. Exclusive breastfeeding for six months offers a lot more protection. For the mother, breastfeeding helps the uterus get back down to size, bonding with the baby, releases a hormone called oxytocin that helps the mother feel calm and connected to the baby, and lowers the risk of breast cancer, ovarian cancer, osteoporosis, diabetes, and cardiovascular disease.

Nutrition

Nutrition is the process of taking in food and converting it into energy and other vital nutrients required for proper functioning, health, and growth in life. In the biochemical and physiological process of nutrition, organisms utilize (metabolize) nutrients such as carbohydrates, fat, protein, vitamins, minerals and roughage to create energy and chemical structures, supporting life. Nutritional stages are ingestion, digestion, absorption, transport, assimilation, and excretion. Failure to obtain the required amount of nutrients causes malnutrition. The nutrition aspect of this chapter has some connection to the previous Chapter 11 on Obesity

DOI: 10.1201/9781003438366-12

and Physical Activity, but care has been taken to separate these wherever possible.

REVIEWS OF EVIDENCE

There were 24 reviews on breastfeeding and nine on nutrition. Several reviews of breastfeeding focused on low- and middle-income countries, and this focus was again prominent in the reviews of nutrition.

Breastfeeding

Twenty-six peer-reviewed publications were examined by Chapman et al. (2010) in a systematic review, studying effect on rates of breastfeeding initiation, duration, exclusivity, and maternal and child health outcomes. The overwhelming majority of evidence showed that peer counselors improved rates of breastfeeding initiation, duration, and exclusivity. Peer counseling interventions were also shown to significantly decrease the incidence of infant diarrhea and significantly increase the duration of lactational amenorrhea. Ingram et al. (2010) examined the effect of antenatal peer support on rates of breastfeeding initiation in a systematic review of five databases from 1980 to 2009. They selected 11 studies. Seven of these evaluated universal peer support and four targeted antenatal peer support. Universal antenatal peer support did not appear to improve rates of breastfeeding initiation, but targeted antenatal peer support could be beneficial.

A meta-synthesis of 31 qualitative studies in peer-reviewed journals was undertaken by Schmied et al. (2011) between 1990 and 2007, including studies of formal or 'created' peer and professional support for breastfeeding women but excluding studies of family or informal support. Four categories included a total of 20 themes. Support for breastfeeding occurred along a continuum from authentic presence at one end (perceived as effective support) to disconnected encounters at the other (perceived as ineffective or even discouraging and counterproductive). Person-centered communication skills in supporting women to breastfeed were important. Seven databases were searched by Demirtas (2012) between 1995 and 2011, including 38 papers. Strategies to support breastfeeding included collaboration with community and family members; confidence building; appropriate ratio of staffing levels; development of communication skills; and 'closing the gap' in inequalities in health. Mothers benefited when their self-efficacy was supported, and they felt capable and empowered. Support needed to be tailored to their individual needs.

Kaunonen et al. (2012) conducted a systematic literature review from three databases 2000–2008 but only of English-speaking countries. Individual support and education were used most during pregnancy and hospitalization, while peer support was strongly associated with the postnatal period. Continuous professional and peer support together were effective in ensuring the continuation of breastfeeding. Professionals required breastfeeding education as well as the support of their organizations in this work. A systematic review and meta-analysis by Shakya et al. (2017) in six databases had three outcome variables: exclusive breastfeeding duration, breastfeeding within the first hour of life, and pre-lacteal feeding. Meta-analyses of RCTs (randomized controlled trials) and quasi-experimental studies were conducted, and 47 articles selected. In low- and middle-income countries, peer support increased exclusive breastfeeding at three, five, and six months. In high-income countries, however, peer support only increased exclusive breastfeeding at three months. In low- and middle-income countries, peer support increased the initiation of breastfeeding within the first hour of life and decreased the risk of pre-lacteal feeding.

Whitford et al. (2017) investigated breastfeeding in women who had given birth to more than one infant, which could be more challenging. The extra demands on the mother of frequent suckling and coordinating the needs of more than one infant could lead to delayed initiation or early cessation. Three databases were searched and ten RCTs extracted, resulting in ten trials (23 reports) involving 5,787 women. None of the interventions were specifically designed for women with more than one infant and outcomes were not reported separately for each infant. The authors found no evidence about the effectiveness of breastfeeding education and support for women with twins or higher order multiples, or the most effective way to provide education and support. Breastfeeding support interventions enabling mothers to practice breastfeeding for six months were studied by Kim et al. (2018). Six databases were searched for RCTs from 2000 to 2017 and 27 articles included. The effectiveness of interventions was highly significant. In addition, a hospital initiative intervention, a combined intervention, a professional provider led intervention, having a protocol available for the provider training program, and implementation during both the prenatal and postnatal periods increased the rate of breast feeding.

An overview of peer support in the U.K. was the goal of Grant et al. (2018). National Health Service (NHS) organizations (n = 177) were surveyed, and 136 responses received (out of 696, response rate 19.5%). Breastfeeding peer supporters were available in 56% of NHS organization areas and breastfeeding support groups in 89% of NHS organization areas. However, areas were often large, and women might still face issues accessing peer supporters or breastfeeding support groups. Coverage within areas was variable. The provision of training and ongoing supervision, and peer supporter roles, varied significantly between services. One quarter of respondents stated that breastfeeding peer support was not accessed by mothers from poorer social backgrounds. Buckland et al. (2020) conducted a systematic review that explored interventions to increase exclusive breastfeeding among young mothers in high-income countries. Nine databases were searched and nine studies included (eight in the United States). Most studies included a combination of strategies, peer counseling being the most common. No significant difference was detected in the rate of exclusive breastfeeding. This review was limited by the relatively few studies which met the inclusion criteria and the small sample sizes of included studies.

A systematic review by Camacho and Hussain (2020) searched two databases and focused on costs. Only four papers were included, which generally indicated that interventions were cost-effective. Peer support for breastfeeding was associated with longer duration of exclusivity with costs ranging from GBP £19–£107 per additional month. Chepkirui et al. (2020) conducted a scoping review, searching five databases and including 18 articles, of which only five were from low-income countries. Most of the supporters were employed ($n = 10$) compared to volunteers ($n = 3$) and support was mainly one-to-one ($n = 11$) rather than group support. Thirteen studies reported positive breastfeeding outcomes. A systematic review was conducted by Rodríguez-Gallego et al. (2021) from 2015 to 2020 in six databases and 13 articles included. The most successful strategies to support and maintain breastfeeding during postpartum were those that combined peer support with counseling by a health professional. Hoy et al. (2021) conducted a scoping review of peer support in high-income countries, including 24 articles describing 12 interventions. Most interventions were designed and implemented with a top-down approach. Evaluation findings indicated interventions were capable of increasing initiation, duration, and exclusivity of breastfeeding. Positive psychosocial benefits for mothers and positive health impacts for infants were reported.

Seven databases were searched by Chang et al. (2022), including 23 papers. Breastfeeding peer support increased women's self-esteem and confidence in breastfeeding while reducing social isolation. Peer supporters valued the experience, which gave them a sense of purpose and confidence, and felt good about helping the women they supported. Women appreciated peer supporters who were caring, spent time with them, shared experiences, provided realistic information, practical and emotional support. Yas et al. (2023) also noted that adolescent mothers breastfed less than adult mothers. Nine databases were searched and 11 articles selected. A meta-analysis showed highly significant results ($p = 0.001$). A scoping review by Ummah et al. (2023) searched three databases and included nine studies reporting the effect of breastfeeding peer education. Reicher and Spatz (2024) searched four databases from 2013 to 2023 and included ten studies. Eight were qualitative, one was an RCT, and one used mixed methods. Parents found comfort in online support groups because they normalized more unique feeding practices and offered a space to provide and receive encouragement.

Low- and Middle-Income Countries

For a systematic review, Jolly et al. (2012) searched five databases from 1980 to 2011 for RCTs. Effects were estimated for studies according to context (high-income countries, low- or middle-income countries), intensity (< 5 and ≥ 5 planned contacts), and timing of peer support (postnatal period with or without antenatal care). Peer support had a significantly greater effect in low- or middle-income countries, reducing the risk of not breastfeeding at all by 30% compared to 7% in high-income countries. Similarly, the risk of non-exclusive breast feeding decreased significantly more in low- or middle-income countries. Peer support had a greater effect on breastfeeding when given at higher intensity and only delivered in the postnatal period.

Sudfeld et al. (2012) also examined the effect of peer support on duration of exclusive breastfeeding in low- and middle-income countries, searching three databases to 2012 and including 11 RCTs. They noted significant differences in training methods, peer visit schedules, and outcome ascertainment. Peer support significantly decreased the risk of discontinuing breastfeeding as compared to controls, including in low-birth-weight infants. Traditional methods of systematic review were ill-equipped to explore the heterogeneity, complexity, and context influences on effectiveness in low-income countries, according to Trickey et al. (2018). Transferable theories to inform design emerged, in seven categories: (a) congruence with local infant feeding norms, (b) integration with the existing system of health care, (c) overcoming practical and emotional barriers to access, (d) ensuring friendly, competent and proactive peers, (e) facilitating authentic peer–mother interactions, (f) motivating peers to ensure positive within-intervention amplification, and (g) ensuring positive legacy and maintenance of gains.

Olufunlayo et al. (2019) conducted a systematic review of various interventions on breastfeeding up to six months in low- and middle-income countries. Three databases were searched and 67 studies from 30 countries included. At six months, intervention group infants were more likely to be exclusively breastfed than controls. Larger effects were obtained from interventions delivered by a combination of professional and laypersons, in interventions spanning antenatal and post-natal periods and when intensity was between four and eight contacts/sessions. A synthesis of evidence on existing breastfeeding support packages for infants under six months in low- and middle-income countries was conducted by Rana et al. (2021). Five databases were searched to 2018, including 41 studies from 22 countries. Among all interventions, breastfeeding counseling ($n = 6$) and education ($n = 6$) support packages showed the most positive effect on breastfeeding practices, followed by peer support ($n = 3$).

Yang et al. (2024) conducted a qualitative systematic review aiming to synthesize qualitative findings on mothers' experiences of breastfeeding peer support to provide evidence for optimizing peer support services. Ten databases were searched until January 2023 and 15 articles extracted. The articles reviewed mostly originated from developed countries. Mothers perceived that peer support had a positive impact on breastfeeding. To improve the effectiveness of peer support in promoting breastfeeding, it was important to consider the individual needs of each mother.

Nutrition

A systematic review specifically on peer education/counseling in nutrition and health outcomes among Latinos was conducted by Perez-Escamilla et al. (2008). The authors reviewed 22 articles on experimental or quasi-experimental studies. Peer education had a positive influence on diabetes self-management and breastfeeding outcomes, as well as on general nutrition knowledge and dietary intake behaviors among Latinos. Nelson and Nickols-Richardson (2014) and Nickols-Richardson et al. (2014) studied school-based peer nutrition education interventions for students aged 2–19 years from 1977 to 2013, examining 15 articles. Some evidence showed peer education improved attitudes, self-efficacy, and perceptions related to a healthy lifestyle. However, evidence of impact on physical measurements was scarce.

Yip et al. (2016) also studied school-based, peer-led nutrition education initiatives, searching four databases but only for North American studies 2000–2013, including 17 articles. Common outcome measures included healthy eating knowledge ($n = 5$), self-efficacy or attitudes toward healthy eating ($n = 13$), dietary measures ($n = 9$), and body mass index ($n = 4$), all of which tended to improve because of the programs. The long-term maintenance of positive impacts was a challenge. A systematic review assessed the effectiveness of peer support for encouraging dietary behavior change in adults (Moore et al., 2017). Five databases were searched and 26 studies included, mostly from the USA. Most studies used group-based peer support. Dietary outcomes measured included dietary pattern, fruit and vegetable intake, fat intake, and intake of other nutrients. Measurement of dietary change was largely based on self-report tools rather than objective measures of actual change. More studies reported a positive effect of peer support on dietary change (23%) or mixed effects (46%), than studies that did not find an effect (31%).

Janmohamed et al. (2020) synthesized the evidence for the effectiveness of nutrition-specific intervention delivery platforms for improving nutrition outcomes in low- and middle-income countries. A systematic search from 1997 to 2018 resulted in the inclusion of 83 studies. Community health worker home visits increased early initiation of breastfeeding and exclusive breastfeeding. Mother/peer groups were effective for improving children's minimum dietary diversity and minimum meal frequency. Studies using both home visit and group methods showed positive results. Complementary feeding could reduce the risk of malnutrition and was especially important in Asian and African countries (Haque et al., 2023). The effectiveness of peer counseling in Asian and African countries (Bangladesh, India, Nepal, and Somalia) was examined, searching seven databases from 2000 to 2021 and including six studies, of which three studies were RCTs and three quasi-experimental. Peer counseling was effective in improving timely initiation of complementary feeding, minimum meal frequency, and minimum dietary diversity in all studies.

Kulandaivelu et al. (2023) conducted a scoping review of social media interventions for nutrition education among adolescents, searching five databases and including 28 papers. Fourteen interventions used homegrown social media platforms, eight used Facebook, and two used Instagram. Engagement with interventions was variable, but high engagement was not required to elicit significant improvements in dietary behaviors. Tailoring interventions, offering practical content, meaningful peer support, and involving families and communities facilitated successful interventions. Thus, social media interventions for adolescent nutrition were acceptable and improved nutritional outcomes. Diseases in Papua New Guinea were studied by Chen et al. (2024), who searched four databases and included 23 papers, of which 12 were developing personal skills programs. Enablers included community involvement, cultural appropriateness, strong leadership, and the use of mobile health technologies. Barriers included limited resources and funding and a lack of central leadership to drive ongoing implementation.

SINGLE STUDIES

Number of Single Studies

There were 101 single studies of breastfeeding (39 from developing countries and 62 from developed countries) and 30 single studies of nutrition (12 from developing countries–40%–and 17 from developed countries). As the number of reviews was so large, we will not examine any single studies other than the implementation exemplar (which is rather long). The full list of single studies is available online.

SPECIFIC PROGRAM

Nankunda et al. (2010) reported on a peer counseling program for breast-feeding in Uganda, where 98% of children are ever breastfed, but exclusive breastfeeding levels remain low.

Effectiveness

Twelve women were identified by their communities, one from each of 12 clusters. They were trained for six days and followed up for one year while they counseled mothers. Their knowledge and attitudes toward exclusive breastfeeding were assessed before and immediately after training and ten months into peer counseling. Observations, field notes, and records of interactions with peer counselors were used to record experiences from this intervention. The communities were receptive to peer counseling and women participated willingly. After training and ten-month follow-up, their knowledge and attitude to exclusive breastfeeding improved. All were retained in the study and mothers accepted them in their homes. They checked for mothers several times if they missed them on the first attempt. Involving the communities in selection helped to identify reliable breastfeeding peer counselors who were acceptable to mothers.

Implementation

In Uganda, most women initiate breastfeeding, but many introduce other feeds early, leading to low levels of exclusive breastfeeding by the age of six months. Giving pre-lacteal feeds has also been reported as common in Uganda. Most reasons for giving pre-lacteal feeds and early complementary feeds result from misconceptions about the infant's needs. Some women give their infants complementary foods early because they think they do not have enough breast milk or believe that breast milk alone is not sufficient for their babies' nutritional needs.

This chapter describes establishing individual peer counseling including training and retaining peer counselors for exclusive breastfeeding. It is a multicenter, community-randomized trial in Burkina Faso, Uganda, Zambia, and South Africa. The Uganda site is in Mbale district, Eastern Uganda, which has a population of about 720,000. The study was carried out in the urban Mbale municipality and the rural Bungokho County. The majority are Bagisu who use Lumasaba as their main language, while some minority tribes (Iteso, Baganda, and Bagweri) speak different languages but are also able to understand Lumasaba.

The intervention of peer counseling for exclusive breastfeeding was set up in 12 clusters, nine rural and three urban, each with an estimated population of 1,000 inhabitants, expected to provide 35 babies in a year given a birth rate of 3.5%. Each rural cluster consisted of one to three villages combined, depending on the village population size. Two of the three urban clusters comprised densely populated areas of Mbale town with poor housing and overcrowding.

Identification of Peer Counselors

The study team invited the village local council chairpersons to a meeting where they were informed about the study. Each of the leaders subsequently organized a meeting with women in their respective villages (12 meetings). At these meetings, the study team explained to the women what the study was about and the need to identify one of their numbers to be trained as a peer counselor for breastfeeding. The women proposed two to three candidates who were then interviewed by the study team. To be selected, a woman had to be aged between 18 and 45 years, and to be resident in the area with no plans of leaving the area within two years. She had to have a good reputation in the community. Further, she had to be literate and numerate in the local language, willing to participate in the study including a one-week residential training, and to undertake home visits in order to help women breastfeed their babies. Previous personal experience of breastfeeding was an additional inclusion criterion. The selected woman was announced as the peer counselor.

Training of Peer Counselors

The 12 selected women were given six days of training using simplified materials based on the WHO Breastfeeding Counselling Course (https://www.who.int/publications/i/item/WHO-CDR-93.3-5). The methods used included lectures, small group discussions, plenary discussions, role plays, and hands-on practice with mothers who had just delivered at Mbale Regional Referral Hospital. During the clinical practice sessions, the women were observed counseling the mothers and helping them with positioning and attachment of their babies at the breast. The gaps identified in their knowledge and skills were addressed by the study team to improve their skills. The languages used in training were English and the two local languages commonly used in the area, Lumasaba and Luganda. The procedures of the study were also taught: how to complete the peer counselor visit forms and record information at each visit. This information included dates of visits, duration of session, and a checklist of topics discussed with the mothers. The proper timing of peer counselor visits and the key messages to share with the mothers during different visits were emphasized. All 12 peer counselors completed the training and started supporting mothers in their villages with breastfeeding. All trainers had earlier been trained as trainers using the La Leche League training curriculum (https://laleche.org.uk/product/beginning-breastfeeding-course/). The supervisory team comprised the lead trainer and a social worker who was trained with the peer counselors and given further training for supervising the peer counselors.

Key Messages

Antenatal visit:

- Skin-to-skin contact between baby and mother after birth
- Early initiation of breastfeeding within one hour
- Colostrum is good for the baby
- Give no pre-lacteal feeds to baby
- Frequent breastfeeding increases breast milk production
- Baby should empty one breast before changing to another breast
- Breastfeed exclusively for six months

Subsequent visits:

- Good attachment and positioning
- Frequent breastfeeding increases breast milk production
- Baby should empty one breast before changing to another breast
- How to handle a crying baby
- Expressing and storing breast milk
- Normal stools and normal urination
- Breastfeed exclusively for six months
- Mother should eat properly and practice good hygiene.

Characteristics of Peer Counselors

The women were aged 25–40 years (average 34). All had attained at least seven years of formal education. Eleven were married, and most were full-time subsistence farmers and child carers. All had breastfed their babies except one who had not yet had a baby of her own. More than half had fed their babies according to the WHO guidelines.

Impact of Training

Before starting the training, the women were given a non-standardized pre-test. This included both open-ended and closed questions on their knowledge about exclusive breastfeeding, as well as questions assessing their attitudes to and beliefs about exclusive breastfeeding. This highlighted problem areas concerning knowledge about breastfeeding. The same questions were repeated at post-test immediately after training and again ten months into the peer counseling process (available in the original article). The demographic characteristics of each peer counselor and her practices in feeding her youngest child were obtained. During the training, the women's participation in training activities was observed, and their understanding of the course content was assessed.

Peer Counseling Intervention

The peer counselors were to visit each mother at least five times, the first visit occurring when a mother was about seven months pregnant. The remaining visits were made during the first, fourth, seventh, and tenth weeks after delivery. Mothers with breastfeeding problems were given extra visits. Extra visits were also given if a mother called the peer counselor for additional assistance.

Supervision

The key follow-up activities were supervision visits by the supervisory team and monthly meetings between this team and all the peer counselors. The supervisory team visited each peer counselor at least once every two weeks. They checked visit forms for completeness. Any achievements and challenges were discussed, and a way forward was agreed. Interesting experiences were noted by the supervisory team for sharing with the whole group at the subsequent monthly meeting. The supervisory team observed each peer counselor counseling one mother once a month. After she had finished a counseling session and left the mother's compound, the supervisor gave her feedback on her performance. The peer counselors were invited to monthly meetings with the supervisors at the study office. At these meetings, they presented and discussed reports about their activities, achievements, and challenges.

Remuneration

The peer counselors were provided with a small allowance of about 10% of a teacher's monthly salary (around US$20 per month). This amount was agreed upon by both the study team and the peer counselors.

Monitoring

The peer counseling process was monitored. Each visit was recorded on a form shown to the supervisors. The supervisory team made records of visits to peer counselors, the observed counseling sessions, and the field observations. Minutes of the monthly meetings were recorded as well as the topics discussed at different meetings.

Implications For Scaling-Up

Peer counseling interventions in similar settings should consider:

- Using existing community leadership channels help to gain confidence of the community
- Sensitization of the community about the study at the onset of the study to avoid undue expectations, which cannot be satisfied by the available resources
- Understanding the social dynamics and power structures at the family and community level helps to avoid collisions during the study period
- Understanding who the other stakeholders concerned with infant feeding are to involve them in the peer counseling process
- Stay clear of other projects/political rallies with different goals and possible other remuneration schemes.
- Adequate training of the peer counselors before they embark on counseling mothers, as they are assessed by the mothers and accepted depending on the quality of what they deliver
- Continuous support supervision of the peer counselors by the study team helps them to improve their knowledge and skills as well as boosting their morale
- The peer counselors need to be allowed some degree of flexibility regarding timing of visits for them to easily fit them into their regular schedules

- Maintaining an allowance for the peer counselors helps to keep them well motivated to continue helping mothers
- To plan the practical part of the peer counseling, there is a need for a thorough understanding of the behaviors and practices of the community women after childbirth, for example, where they go and what they do.

REFERENCES

Buckland, C., Hector, D., Kolt, G. S., Fahey, P., & Arora, A. (2020). Interventions to promote exclusive breastfeeding among young mothers: A systematic review and meta-analysis. *International Breastfeeding Journal, 15*(1), 1–14. https://doi.org/10.1186/s13006-020-00340-6

Camacho, E. M., & Hussain, H. (2020). Cost-effectiveness evidence for strategies to promote or support breastfeeding: A systematic search and narrative literature review. *BMC Pregnancy and Childbirth, 20*(1), 757. https://doi.org/10.1186/s12884-020-03460-3

Chang, Y. S., Beake, S., Kam, J., Lok, K. Y. W., & Bick, D. (2022). Views and experiences of women, peer supporters and healthcare professionals on breastfeeding peer support: A systematic review of qualitative studies. *Midwifery, 108*, 103299. https://doi.org/10.1016/j.midw.2022.103299

Chapman, D. J., Morel, K., Anderson, A. K., Damio, G., & Pérez-Escamilla, R. (2010). Breastfeeding peer counseling: From efficacy through scale-up. *Journal of Human Lactation, 26*(3), 314–326. https://doi.org/10.1177/0890334410369481

Chen, J., Davies, A., Tran, P., Gronau, R., Rangan, A., & Allman-Farinelli, M., et al. (2024). Health and nutrition promotion programs in papua new Guinea: A scoping review. *Nutrients, 16*, 1999. https://doi.org/10.3390/nu16131999

Chepkirui, D., Nzinga, J., Jemutai, J., Tsofa, B., Jones, C., & Mwangome, M. (2020). A scoping review of breastfeeding peer support models applied in hospital settings. *International Breastfeeding Journal, 15*, 95. https://doi.org/10.1186/s13006-020-00331-7

Demirtas, B. (2012). Strategies to support breastfeeding: A review. *International Nursing Review, 59*(4), 474–481. https://doi.org/10.1111/j.1466-7657.2012.01017.x

Grant, A., McEwan, K., Tedstone, S., Greene, G., Copeland, L., & Hunter, B., et al. (2018). Availability of breastfeeding peer support in the United Kingdom: A cross-sectional study. *Maternal and Child Nutrition, 14*, e12476. https://doi.org/10.1111/mcn.12476

Haque, N. B., Mihrshahi, S., & Haider, R. (2023). Peer counselling as an approach to improve complementary feeding practices: A narrative review. *Journal of Health Population and Nutrition, 42*(1), Article Number 60. https://doi.org/10.1186/s41043-023-00408-z

Hoy, S., Harrison, J., Craig, A., & Lafrenière, G. (2021). The "calm in the storm": A scoping review of in-hospital peer support breastfeeding interventions. *Diversity of Research in Health Journal, 4,* 65–86. https://doi.org/10.28984/drhj.v4i1.319

Ingram, L., MacArthur, C., Khan, K., Deeks, J. J., & Jolly, K. (2010). Effect of antenatal peer support on breastfeeding initiation: A systematic review. *Canadian Medical Association Journal, 182*(16), 1739–1746. https://doi.org/10.1503/cmaj.091729

Janmohamed, A., Sohani, N., Lassi, Z. S., & Bhutta, Z. A. (2020). The effects of community home visit and peer group nutrition intervention delivery platforms on nutrition outcomes in low and middle-income countries: A systematic review and meta-analysis. *Nutrients, 12,* 440. https://doi.org/10.3390/nu12020440

Jolly, K., Ingram, L., Khan, K. S., Deeks, J. J., Freemantle, N., & MacArthur, C. (2012). Systematic review of peer support for breastfeeding continuation: Metaregression analysis of the effect of setting, intensity, and timing. *BMJ, 344,* d8287. https://doi.org/10.1136/bmj.d8287

Kaunonen, M., Hannula, L., & Tarkka, M. (2012). A systematic review of peer support interventions for breastfeeding. *Journal of Clinical Nursing, 21,* 1943–1954. https://doi.org/10.1111/j.1365-2702.2012.04071.x

Kim, K., Park, S., Oh, J., Kim, J., & Ahn, S. (2018). Interventions promoting exclusive breastfeeding up to six months after birth: A systematic review and meta-analysis of randomized controlled trials. *International Journal of Nursing Studies, 80,* 94–105. https://doi.org/10.1016/j.ijnurstu.2018.01.004

Kulandaivelu, Y., Hamilton, J., Banerjee, A., Gruzd, A., Patel, B., & Stinson, J. (2023). Social media interventions for nutrition education among adolescents: Scoping review. *JMIR Pediatrics and Parenting, 6,* e36132. https://doi.org/10.2196/36132

Moore, S. E., McEvoy, C. T., McKinley, M. C., & Woodside, J. V. (2017). The effectiveness of peer support in encouraging dietary behaviour change in adults: A systematic review. *Proceedings of the Nutrition Society, 76*(OCE3), E111. Irish Section Meeting, 21–23 June 2017. What governs what we eat? https://doi.org/10.1017/S0029665117001847

Nankunda, J., Tylleskär, T., Ndeezi, G., Semiyaga, N., & Tumwine, J. K. (2010). Establishing individual peer counselling for exclusive breastfeeding in Uganda: Implications for scaling-up. *Maternal and Child Nutrition, 6,* 53–66. https://doi.org/10.1111/j.1740-8709.2009.00187.x

Nelson, S. A., & Nickols-Richardson, S. M. (2014). A systematic review of peer nutrition education in childhood and adolescence. *Health Behavior and Policy Review, 1*(4), 247–264. https://doi.org/10.14485/HBPR.1.4.1

Nickols-Richardson, S. M., Nelson, S. A., & Corbin, M. A. (2014). Peer Nutrition education in childhood and adolescence: Evidence-based guidance for impactful programs. *Journal of Nutrition Education and Behavior, 46*(4), S196. https://www.jneb.org/cms/10.1016/j.jneb.2014.04.211/attachment/a6346c97-3681-44a9-8e4f-9b5f9eb873f1/mmc1.pdf

Olufunlayo, T. F., Roberts, A. A., MacArthur, C., Thomas, N., Odeyemi, K. A., & Price, M., et al. (2019). Improving exclusive breastfeeding in low and middle-income countries: A systematic review. *Maternal and Child Nutrition, 15,* e12788. https://doi.org/10.1111/mcn.12788

Perez-Escamilla, R., Hromi-Fiedler, A., Vega-Lopez, S., Bermudez-Millan, A., & Segura-Perez, S. (2008). Impact of peer nutrition education on dietary behaviors and health outcomes among Latinos: A systematic literature review. *Journal of Nutrition Education and Behavior*, *40*(4), 208–225. https://doi.org/10.1016/j.jneb.2008.03.011

Rana, R., McGrath, M., Sharma, E., Gupta, P., & Kerac, M. (2021). Effectiveness of breastfeeding support packages in low- and middle-income countries for infants under six months: A systematic review. *Nutrients*, *13*, 681. https://doi.org/10.3390/nu13020681

Reicher, H. K., & Spatz, D. L. (2024). Breastfeeding, chestfeeding, and lactating parents' experiences with online support groups: An integrative review. *Journal of Midwifery & Women's Health*, 69, 531–542. https://doi.org/10.1111/jmwh.13618

Rodríguez-Gallego, I., Leon-Larios, F., Corrales-Gutierrez, I., & González-Sanz, J. D. (2021). Impact and effectiveness of group strategies for supporting breastfeeding after birth: A systematic review. *International Journal of Environmental Research and Public Health*, *18*, 2550. https://doi.org/10.3390/ijerph18052550

Schmied, V., Beake, S., Sheehan, A., McCourt, C., & Dykes, F. (2011). Women's perceptions and experiences of breastfeeding support: A metasynthesis. *Birth*, *38*(1), 49–60. https://doi.org/10.1111/j.1523-536X.2010.00446.x

Shakya, P., Kunieda, M. K., Koyama, M., Rai, S. S., Miyaguchi, M., & Dhakal, S., et al. (2017). Effectiveness of community-based peer support for mothers to improve their breastfeeding practices: A systematic review and meta-analysis. *PLoS ONE*, *12*(5), e0177434. https://doi.org/10.1371/journal.pone.0177434

Sudfeld, C. R., Fawzi, W. W., & Lahariya, C. (2012). Peer support and exclusive breastfeeding duration in low and middle-income countries: A systematic review and meta-analysis. *PLoS ONE*, *7*(9), e45143. https://doi.org/10.1371/journal.pone.0045143

Trickey, H., Thomson, G., Grant, A., Sanders, J., Mann, M., & Murphy, S., et al. (2018). A realist review of one-to-one breastfeeding peer support experiments conducted in developed country settings. *Maternal and Child Nutrition*, *14*, e12559. https://doi.org/10.1111/mcn.12559

Ummah, F., Rosida, L., & Putri, A. K. (2023). Breastfeeding education: A scoping review. *Malaysian Journal of Medicine and Health Sciences*, *19*(2), 293–302. https://doi.org/10.47836/mjmhs19.2.41

Whitford, H. M., Wallis, S. K., Dowswell, T., West, H. M., & Renfrew, M. J. (2017). Breastfeeding education and support for women with twins or higher order multiples. *Cochrane Database of Systematic Reviews*, *2*, Article Number CD012003. https://doi.org/10.1002/14651858.CD012003.pub2

Yang, Y., Liu, H., Cui, X., & Meng, J. (2024). Mothers' experiences and perceptions of breastfeeding peer support: A qualitative systematic review. *International Breastfeeding Journal*, *19*(1), 7. https://doi.org/10.1186/s13006-024-00614-3

Yas, A., Abdollahi, M., Khadivzadeh, T., & Zahra Karimi, F. (2023). Investigating the effect of supportive interventions on initiation of breastfeeding, exclusive breastfeeding, and continuation of breastfeeding in adolescent mothers: A systematic review and meta-analysis. *Breastfeeding Medicine*, *18*(3), 198–211. https://doi.org/10.1089/bfm.2022.0219

Yip, C., Gates, M., Gates, A., & Hanning, R. M. (2016). Peer-Led nutrition education programs for school-aged youth: A systematic review of the literature. *Health Education Research*, *31*(1), 82–97. https://doi.org/10.1093/her/cyv063

Prisons 13

DEFINITION

A prison is a building in which people are legally held for a period as a punishment for a crime they have committed or while they are awaiting trial. In this chapter, we are considering peer interventions actually within prisons, rather than also considering peer interventions for released prisoners returning to the community (although there is a fair amount of literature on this latter topic as well). Of course, this chapter seems out of place in this book, as it refers to a location rather than medical conditions or wellbeing, but much of the work here is about HIV/AIDS prevention and treatment (also see Chapter 3), drug abuse (also see Chapter 9), and suicide prevention (also see Chapter 7).

REVIEWS OF EVIDENCE

There were 14 reviews of evidence, mostly general reviews of peer intervention in all conditions. In addition, there were two reviews of peer intervention in HIV/AIDS, one on self-injury and one on sexual offenders.

General

The earliest classic review was by Devilly et al. (2005), who explored the theoretical underpinnings of peer programs, followed by a general overview of the then scarce empirical research on correctional peer programs in the areas of HIV/AIDS and health education, drug and alcohol abuse, sexual assault/offending, prison orientation, and suicide/violence prevention. The study then focused on the difficulties of implementing such programs, as well as their appeal.

DOI: 10.1201/9781003438366-13

The authors concluded that while preliminary reports of offender–peer programs were positive, controlled research was lacking. They provided a guide to effectively implement and evaluate peer programs.

By 2011, Wright et al. (2011) were able to systematically review the literature, searching six databases and including 46 articles, of which only ten were finally included in the review. They found that peer education in prisons could have an impact on attitudes, knowledge, and behavioral intentions regarding HIV risk behavior. Findings were inconclusive for illicit drug use and injecting. There was a paucity of research on mental ill health, obesity, diet, smoking, or self-management of physical diseases. A further systematic review in 2014 by South et al. (2014) searched 20 databases and included 57 studies. Only one study considered cost-effectiveness; most were of poor methodological quality. Evidence suggested that peer education interventions were effective at reducing risky behaviors and that peer support services had a positive effect on recipients. The strongest evidence came from the Listener scheme. Being a peer deliverer was associated with positive effects across all intervention types. Peer-led education was more cost-effective than professionally led education for the prevention of HIV infection.

Bagnall et al. (2015) offered a further systematic review, searching 19 databases from 1985 to 2012 and including 57 studies, mostly of poor methodological quality. Evidence suggested that peer education interventions were effective at reducing risky behaviors. Peer support services were acceptable within the prison environment and had a positive effect on recipients, practically or emotionally. Being a peer deliverer was associated with positive effects. Expert views of peer-based interventions for prisoner health were the focus of Woodall et al. (2015). Individuals with recognized professional expertise from various sectors (including ex-prisoners) contributed to an expert symposium. Peer interventions had both positive and negative impacts. They could impact positively on health outcomes, but effects were more well-defined for peer deliverers. Supervisory processes for peer workers needed to be considered. South et al. (2016) then offered a qualitative synthesis of positive and negative outcomes from 33 studies. Themes were grouped into four thematic categories: peer recruitment training and support; organizational support; prisoner relationships; prison life. There was consistent qualitative evidence on the need for organizational support within the prison to ensure smooth implementation. Alongside reported benefits of peer delivery, some reasons for non-utilization of services by other prisoners were found.

Further work from South et al. (2017) sought to develop a typology for peer education and peer support delivered by prisoners. Peer interventions were grouped into four modes: peer education, peer support, peer mentoring, and bridging roles. Warren and Nadia (2017) conducted a systematic literature review, which retrieved articles on prisoner caregiving and the main themes were identified. The main themes were the benefits of prisoner care-giving; training needs; and the organizational implications of implementing prisoner caregiving. The role of prisoner caregiver was increasingly recognized as important and was associated with several benefits to individual prisoners and the prison community. However, further training was required for prisoner caregivers. Elisha (2022) focused on the role of the" wounded healer", as exemplified by former addicts and prisoners who desisted from crime and recovered through the practice of peer mentoring. Incarcerated people employed in peer-based rehabilitation roles could benefit by experiencing accomplishments and developing an increasing sense of ability and self-worth. Additional benefits included acquiring a new meaning and purpose in life, the development of a new self-identity, increasing feelings of belonging and satisfaction from life, and a stronger commitment to avoid crime.

Incarcerated populations are more likely to suffer from mental health and substance use disorders and from violent and self-harm behaviors than the general population (McCrary et al., 2022). Eighty-five percent of incarcerated individuals were either struggling with active substance abuse disorders or were under the influence of alcohol and/or drugs at the time of their crime. Despite 1.5 million inmates meeting clinical criteria for substance abuse in the USA, only 168,000 received treatment. Additionally, one-third of the 2.3 million persons in prison in the USA had a diagnosis of a mental illness. The risk of opioid overdose in the first two weeks following an individual's release from prison was 40 times higher than for the general population. Peer support was a proven resource to address the demands in correctional and community settings to support recovery. Peer support had proved to be effective for a range of emotional, informational, and instrumental supports–including an improved sense of wellbeing. However, peer support focused on healing practices that were strengths-based, holistic, trauma-informed, and person-centered. It could be challenging to foster these attributes in a corrections environment, which was punitive by design, relied on control, and could induce or trigger trauma.

HIV/AIDS

Valera et al. (2017) noted that HIV prevalence in correctional populations was approximately five times that of the general adult population. A systematic review from 1980 to 2014 examined the question of HIV prevention and interventions to reduce inmate HIV-related risk behaviors in U.S. federal and state prisons, including 27 articles. Research related to peer education in HIV prevention was a key topic. Peer educators' competences was the focus of Anisah et al. (2018), who conducted a literature review from

1997 to 2017, searching three databases and including just seven papers. There were three peer educators' competences for inmates with HIV/AIDS: (i) knowledgeable about HIV and related disease, (ii) good communication skill in educating and interacting in the correctional facilities, and (iii) well-behaved in HIV treatment and prevention, daily life, and learning process support. Peer educators' competences thus involved knowledge, communication, and behaviors.

Self-Injury

Griffiths and Bailey (2015) sought to critically evaluate the evidence for peer support in prisons, in particular its contribution to working with prisoners who self-injure. Studies were excluded if the participants' behavior was explicitly linked to suicidal intent, as the review focused on self-injury as a coping strategy. A total of 23 studies were selected: ten focused on peer support and self-injury. The Listener scheme was the focus of 15 studies. The evidence suggested that prison peer support could be considered on a continuum depending on the different degrees of peer involvement.

Sexual Offenders

Incarcerated sexual offenders receiving peer support were studied by Perrin et al. (2018), who conducted a review. They concluded that there were some promising signs from many qualitative investigations that peer-led roles could bridge many gaps in support within the therapeutic context. It was noted that prisoner-led peer-support initiatives that were characterized by shared problem-solving and reciprocal emotional support could greatly reduce the anxiety prisoners face. Through peer-support, treatment gains might be enhanced and better assimilated into the lives of program-completers.

SINGLE STUDIES

Number of Single Studies

There were 36 single studies. Eleven of these concerned general effects of peer intervention (with one focusing on Aboriginal populations in Australia). Nine of them concerned HV/AIDS (with reports of projects in Siberia,

South Africa, Iran, and Mozambique). Six focused on Hepatitis C. There was one on miscellaneous infectious diseases (Iran) and one on Covid. Turning to mental health, there were two studies (including one from Uganda), two on self-harm and one on suicide prevention. Beyond this, there were two studies on drug abuse (including one in Kirgizstan). Finally, there were two studies on tuberculosis (both from Ethiopia).

Exemplar Single Studies Developed Context

Project Wall Talk was a community-based, peer-led HIV prevention education program implemented in 36 Texas State prison units (Ross et al., 2006). Peer educators completed questionnaires prior to the receipt of a 40-hour intensive training ($N = 590$) and at nine-month follow-up ($N = 257$). Students ($N = 2506$) completed questionnaires pre- and post-receipt of peer educator-led HIV education sessions. Peer educators and their students showed significant increases in HIV-related knowledge. Peer educators showed significant increases in assessment of their skills as educators. Compared with baseline, a significantly greater proportion of peer educators reported ever having had an HIV test. After receiving peer-led education, a significantly larger proportion of students reported they knew their HIV status and more indicated plans to take an HIV test. Additionally, in months 12 and 18 following program implementation, the numbers of HIV tests at the five units that implemented the peer education program were roughly twice that of five matched comparison units.

Hepatitis C virus (HCV) infection is endemic in prison populations. Crowley et al. (2019) focused on peer-supported screening to find hepatitis C cases. A secondary aim was to describe the HCV cascade among those infected including linkage to care and treatment outcomes. In a medium-security Irish male prison housing 538 inmates, a questionnaire, medical records, peer-supported screening, laboratory-based HCV serology tests, and mobile elastography were used. Large numbers of prisoners were involved ($n = 419$). Multiple risk factors for HCV acquisition were identified, including needle sharing (16%) and injecting drug use (33%). On serological testing, 87 (21%) were HCV Ab + ve and 50 (12%) were HCV RNA + ve, of whom 25% showed evidence of liver disease. Eighty-six percent of those with active infection were linked with HCV care, with 33% undergoing or completing treatment. Peer-supported screening was an effective model to find and link prisoners with untreated active HCV infection to HCV care.

Could a brief peer-led problem-support mentor intervention reduce self-harm and violence in an English prison (Perry et al., 2021), given that levels of mental disorder, self-harm, and violent behavior are higher in prisons than outside? Eligible prisoners were trained to become problem-support mentors. Delivery of the intervention took two forms: (i) promotion of the intervention to fellow prisoners, offering support and raising awareness of the intervention but not delivering the skills, and (ii) delivery of the problem-solving therapy skills to selected individual prisoners. Training and intervention adherence was measured using mentor logbooks. An interrupted time series (ITS) design was used on prison data over a 31-month period. Outcomes included self-harm and violent behavior. Data were collected at monthly intervals 16 months pre-, ten months during and six months post-intervention. Qualitative data addressed the acceptability, feasibility, impact, and sustainability of the intervention. A matched-case control study followed people after release to evaluate impact on re-offending up to 16 months later. There was a significant reduction in the incidence of self-harm for those receiving the problem-solving skills. However, no significant reduction was found for incidence of violent behavior.

Exemplar Single Studies Developing Context

A peer-led HIV/AIDS and STI education intervention for prison inmates in South Africa was reported by Sifunda et al. (2008). Using data from three prisons including 263 inmates in a nested experimental design, experimental groups showed higher knowledge of STI and had a more positive intention to reduce risky behavior than the control group in two out of three prisons. Long-term assessment three to six months after release from prison indicated that experimental groups were more positive about sexual communication, self-efficacy, and intention. Groups educated by an HIV-negative educator performed marginally better than groups with an HIV-positive peer educator.

Australian Aboriginal and Torres Strait Islander people experience disproportionately higher rates of sexually transmissible infections (STIs) and bloodborne viruses (BBVs) when compared with the non-Indigenous population (D'Costa et al., 2019). Prevalence of bacterial STIs (such as chlamydia, gonorrhea, trichomonas, and syphilis) in remote areas of Australia are at rates many times higher than for non-Indigenous Australians. Similarly, rates of hepatitis B are disproportionately higher for non-Indigenous people. The Young Deadly STI and BBV Free project was designed to increase the uptake of STI and BBV testing and treatment in young Aboriginal and Torres Strait Islander people. Peer education involved training up to 100 young people across 19 communities in a culturally appropriate and respectful manner on the transmission, testing, and treatment of STIs and BBVs. The trained peer educators then delivered three community education sessions to young people in their respective communities. The peer educator training program contributed to STI and BBV knowledge gains among the peer educators and positively influenced their behavioral intentions and attitudes pertaining to STIs and BBVs. Working with Aboriginal and Torres Strait Islander populations on a highly sensitive, stigmatized topic presented many methodological challenges, particularly in terms of ensuring the collection of reliable evaluation data across geographically remote communities.

Approximately 70% of the world prison population is in low- and middle-income countries, and the prevalence of living with a mental illness diagnosis is high (Kaggwa et al., 2023). People who are incarcerated and have untreated mental health conditions have a high likelihood of self-harming behaviors, violence to others, being physically or sexually victimized, increased rates of recidivism on release, and substance misuse. In Uganda, about 86% of people who are incarcerated live with a mental illness diagnosis, and there are fewer than 20 mental health workers in the correctional system. Uganda has one psychiatrist per one million people. Peer support mental health teams assist in triaging individuals who are suspected of having mental health conditions, act as informal caregivers, and assist them in accessing rehabilitation services. Peer intervention aims to provide traditionally and culturally relevant, reliable, efficient, and cost-effective services. The prison warden chose the peers on the basis of their behaviors and work ethic. The healthcare team trained the peers, who were subsequently assigned to different prison wards. With a train-the-trainer model, experienced peers taught other inexperienced volunteers the various roles required. For example, peers take note of individuals who show deterioration in nutrition intake; have disrupted sleep, communication changes, or unusual aggression patterns. Peers also assist in administering prescribed medication, offer psychological support, and provide food. Regular training needs to develop expertise in mental health screening and enhance early identification of mental health conditions, identify side effects of medications, and participate in monitoring of care to support recovery. The peers should be regularly supervised by qualified mental health workers.

SPECIFIC PROGRAM

The specific paper chosen is by Perrin and Blagden (2016), who examined results from some of the most popular peer intervention programs in prison.

Effectiveness

Perhaps the best recognized peer-support program, which typifies the notion of mutual reciprocity and shared problem-solving, is Alcoholics Anonymous (AA). The AA program encourages recovering alcoholics to share their stories of alcohol addiction and their transitional experiences that led to sobriety. Individuals who are in recovery invite newcomers to share their stories and adopt a mentoring role that involves guiding new members through the Twelve Steps program. Research has consistently revealed positive effects of peer-support programs. There is a need to develop peer interventions that address the problems associated with prisons: high rates of suicide and self-harm; increased levels of violence, drug taking, sexual assault, and bullying; and higher incidences of severe mental illness compared to the general population. The provider of support may also benefit because of the sense-making process involved in giving support and the natural requirement for self-reflection and experiential learning.

The most widely implemented peer-support programs are focused on here: the Listener scheme, the Insiders program, Toe-by-Toe, and the RAPt (Rehabilitation of Addicted Persons Trust) mentoring program. Staff nominated potential participants, and the researchers sent recruitment letters inviting them to participate. A final sample of 17 responded. Eligibility requirements included six months or greater peer volunteer experience, current participation as a volunteer, and at least two years served in prison. The researchers did not offer participants any benefits in exchange for their involvement. The written consent form reiterated the voluntary nature of the study. Participants' crimes were varied, and time spent in prison ranged from two years to over 27 years.

The interview schedule was divided into four sections and covered the following areas:

1. Introductory questions–arrival into prison, initial perceptions of prison life, first encounters with peer-support programs.
2. Views and attitudes regarding peer-support work–initial perceptions of peer-support programs, first involvement, motivations for volunteering.
3. Impact of program involvement on the person–thoughts and feelings regarding peer-support role, exploration of how the role impacted on the individual, and their experiences of imprisonment.
4. Future–views of future in the context of the peer-support role, exploration of how this role has shaped thoughts about future self.

Such programs appeared to have a positive impact in terms of prisoners' views of themselves, their experiences of prison, and their perceptions of life beyond prison. Many respondents made an explicit connection between their peer-support role and reduced offending, and all participants expressed a strong desire to become better people and reintegrate successfully after serving time. Participants from all four programs described their experiences in very positive terms and appeared to be having deep realizations and life changing revelations through their work. In addition to cultivating constructive relationships with prison staff and other prisoners, enjoying personal growth from "doing good", honing positive skills, and keeping busy, participants were also able to have a more generally positive experience of prison life because of their volunteer roles. This experience was a product of gathering positivity and the avoidance of negative labels and destructive stigma. All of these benefits appeared to protect participants against the negativity associated with imprisonment and enabled them.

Implementation

This research took place in five adult male prisons in England, varying in terms of risk category and size.

The Listener Scheme

The Listener scheme was established in 1991 in collaboration with the Samaritans. The Samaritans operate a 24-hour, volunteer hotline across the U.K. and the Republic of Ireland that aims to provide people with an outlet for their emotional distress. The Listener scheme was introduced to help tackle high rates of suicide in prisons. Via the scheme, prisoners suffering distress, despair, and suicidal ideation were able to talk face-to-face about their feelings without judgment and with confidentiality. Prisoners who volunteered to become Listeners went through several weeks of training. Listeners receive a certificate upon completion of their training, and they sign a contract that binds them to the same policies to which Samaritans working in the community also adhere. The Listener team establishes a rota within each prison with the aim of providing a 24-hour service to any prisoner in need (referred to as a "caller").

Callers have two options to contact a Samaritans Listener: 1) they can use a Listener phone in the prison to call a Listener working in a community branch; or 2) they can request to speak to a prison Listener. The majority of prisons in the U.K. now have cordless phones that prisoners can access at any time of the day or night to call Samaritans. This phone is capable only of calling Samaritans branches. When feasible, face-to-face meetings are held in a private environment to allow complete confidentiality. Prison Listeners needing to debrief after a face-to-face meeting (referred to as a call), or needing confidential support, can ask to contact their supporting Samaritans branch by telephone privately. Community volunteers from supporting Samaritans branches attend Listener meetings every two weeks at their allocated prison(s) to provide emotional support for Listeners and to regulate the programs and address any emerging issues.

In addition to listening, members of the program also meet weekly to discuss issues relating to 'caller care' and the general running of the scheme. Furthermore, every prison Listener has a chance to coordinate the program, to be involved in the recruitment and training of new members, and to serve as a representative at safer custody meetings, which address prisoners' rights and safety issues. Prisoners are not paid for becoming Listeners. However, employment in prison is categorized in bands, and each band is associated with different levels of privilege (i.e., extra and improved visits, access to in-cell television and the opportunity to wear one's own clothes). Listeners and Insiders (below) operate within the "red band" and have the highest level of privileges.

The Insiders Program

Initial experiences for new prisoners are traumatic, with around 50% of all prison suicides occurring within the first week of custody. The Insiders program operates in prisons throughout the U.K. and aims to address this problem through reducing anxiety experienced during prisoners' early days in custody. Much of this work involves preventing and addressing bullying issues, and Insiders often promote themselves as anti-bullying mentors. Volunteers also provide basic information and reassurance to new prisoners shortly after their arrival. Insiders are not an alternative to Listeners; they offer a different but complementary peer-support service. As such, it is crucial that Insiders and Listeners understand each other's roles and are able to refer distressed individuals to each other. As with the Listener scheme, the Insiders program also involves the vetting and selection of prisoners who then go through extensive training. Insiders are not bound by the same confidentiality procedures as Listeners and the Insiders program is directed more towards providing practical advice and support. Otherwise, the Insiders program works very similarly to the Listener scheme. Each volunteer not only fulfils a weekly shift commitment but also has the opportunity to run different elements of the program, attend standardization and continual improvement meetings, and represent the program at safer custody meetings.

168 Peer Interventions for Health and Wellbeing

Toe-by-Toe

A 2008 study found that 48% of prisoners had a reading level at or below Level 1 (equivalent to a reading age of 14 to 15), and 65% had a numeracy level at or below Level 1. Additionally, 67% of all prisoners reported being unemployed at the time of imprisonment. A broad body of research suggests that more educated prisoners are less likely to return to prison. Toe-by-Toe is the leading program addressing literacy tutoring in prisons and began in 2000, regulated by the Shannon Trust. This charity's vision is to help prisoners to better engage in their rehabilitation journeys by helping them to read. Once the Shannon Trust has helped to establish a Toe-by-Toe program within a prison, prisoners run the program, supervised and facilitated (in terms of resources, allocation of rooms, and so on) by prison staff via monthly meetings. The foundation of the program lies in a "buddy system" through which older, fluent readers adopt mentor roles and coach lesser able students through a reading program. In prisons, the Shannon Trust trains volunteer prisoners and equips them with materials (principally a Toe-by-Toe manual, https://toe-by-toe.co.uk/what-is-toe-by-toe/). Trained mentors are allocated a small number of mentees, who they meet with for hourly sessions each week. During these sessions, mentees receive support to develop basic literacy skills, aiming to enhance the self-esteem of both mentee and mentor.

RAPt Mentors

RAPt (Rehabilitation of Addicted Persons Trust) provides a range of services in prisons across England and Wales but is particularly well known for its drug and alcohol treatment programs. The RAPt Substance Dependence Treatment Program is an abstinence-based treatment program lasting between 16 and 22 weeks. This program is based on the Twelve Steps principles of AA and Narcotics Anonymous (NA). RAPt trains recovered prisoners (those who have completed the Twelve Steps program) to serve as mentors. These mentors provide support to recovering prisoners through advice, guidance, and effective modeling of pro-social recovery attitudes and behaviors.

REFERENCES

Anisah, R. L., Sofro, M. A. U., & Andriany, M. (2018). Peer educators' competences for inmates with HIV/AIDS: A systematic review. https://doc-pak.undip.ac.id/id/eprint/5970/6/ProceedingBook-C25.pdf#page=15

Bagnall, A., South, J., Hulme, C., Woodall, J., Vinall-Collier, K., & Raine, G., et al. (2015). A systematic review of the effectiveness and cost-effectiveness of peer education and peer support in prisons. *BMC Public Health, 15*, 290. https://doi. org/10.1186/s12889-015-1584-x

Crowley, D., Murtagh, R., Cullen, W., Keevans, M., Laird, E., McHugh, T., et al. (2019). Evaluating peer-supported screening as a hepatitis C case-finding model in prisoners. *Harm Reduction Journal, 16*, 42. https://doi.org/10.1186/ s12954-019-0313-7

D'Costa, B., Lobo, R., Thomas, J., & Ward, J. S. (2019). Evaluation of the young deadly free Peer education training program: Early results, methodological challenges, and learnings for future evaluations. *Fronters in Public Health, 7*, 74. https://doi.org/10.3389/fpubh.2019.00074

Devilly, G. J., Sorbello, L., Eccleston, L., & Ward, T. (2005). Prison-based peer-education schemes. *Aggression and Violent Behavior, 10*, 219–240. https://doi. org/10.1016/j.avb.2003.12.001

Elisha, E. (2022). Inmates in the role of the" wounded healer": The virtues of peer-to-peer programs in prison. *International Journal of Criminology and Sociology, 11*, 11–14. https://doi.org/10.6000/1929-4409.2022.11.02

Griffiths, L., & Bailey, D. (2015). Learning from peer support schemes–can prison listeners support offenders who self-injure in custody? *International Journal of Prisoner Health, 11*(3), 157–168. https://doi.org/10.1108/ IJPH-01-2015-0004

Kaggwa, M. M., Olagunju, A. T., Prat, S., Harms, S., & Chaimowitz, G. (2023). Peer Support mental health teams in correctional settings in Uganda. *The Lancet Psychiatry, 10*(2), 76–79. https://doi.org/10.1016/S2215-0366(22)00431-X

McCrary, H., Etwaroo, E., Marshall, L., Burden, E. St, Pierre, M., & Berkebile, B., et al. (2022). *Peer recovery support services in correctional settings.* Washington, DC: Bureau of Justice Assistance. https://www.drugsandalcohol. ie/36290/1/Altarum_PRSS_in_Correctional_Settings.pdf

Perrin, C., & Blagden, N. (2016). Movements towards desistance via peer-support roles in prison. *The voluntary sector in prisons: Encouraging personal and institutional change*, 115–142. New York: Palgrave Macmillan. https://doi. org/10.1057/978-1-137-54215-1_5

Perrin, C., Frost, A., & Ware, J. B. (2018). The utility of peer-support in enhancing the treatment of incarcerated sexual offenders. *Therapeutic Communities, 39*(1), 35–49. https://doi.org/10.1108/TC-06-2017-0018

Perry, A. E., Waterman, M. G., Dale, V., Moore, K., & House, A. (2021). The effect of a peer-led problem-support mentor intervention on self-harm and violence in prison: An interrupted time series analysis using routinely collected prison data. *EClinicalMedicine, 32*, 100702. https://doi.org/10.1016/j.eclinm.2020.100702

Ross, M. W., Harzke, A. J., Scott, D. P., McCann, K., & Kelley, M. (2006). Outcomes of project wall talk: An HIV/AIDS Peer education program implemented within the Texas state prison system. *AIDS Education and Prevention, 18*(6), 504–517. https://doi.org/10.1521/aeap.2006.18.6.504

Sifunda, S., Reddy, P. S., Braithwaite, R., Stephens, T., Bhengu, S., Ruiter, R. A. C., et al. (2008). The effectiveness of a peer-led HIV/AIDS and STI health education intervention for prison inmates in South Africa. *Health Education & Behavior, 35*(4), 494–508. https://doi.org/10.1177/1090198106294894

South, J., Bagnall, A., Hulme, C., Woodall, J., Longo, R., Dixey, R., et al. (2014). A systematic review of the effectiveness and cost-effectiveness of peer-based interventions to maintain and improve offender health in prison settings. *Health Services and Delivery Research*, 2(35). https://doi.org/10.3310/hsdr02350

South, J., Bagnall, A., & Woodall, J. (2017). Developing a typology for peer education and peer support delivered by prisoners. *Journal of Correctional Health Care*, 23(2), 214–229. https://doi.org/10.1177/1078345817700602

South, J., Woodall, J., Kinsella, K., & Bagnall, A. (2016). A qualitative synthesis of the positive and negative impacts related to delivery of peer-based health interventions in prison settings. *BMC Health Services Research*, 16, 525. https://doi.org/10.1186/s12913-016-1753-3

Valera, P., Chang, Y., & Lian, Z. (2017). HIV risk inside u.S. Prisons: A systematic review of risk reduction interventions conducted in U.S. Prisons. *AIDS Care*, 29(8), 943–952. https://doi.org/10.1080/09540121.2016.1271102

Warren, S., & Nadia, E. (2017). Prisoner peer caregiving: A literature review. *Nursing Standard*, 31(32), 44–51. https://doi.org/10.7748/ns.2017.e10468

Woodall, J., South, J., Dixey, R., de Viggiani, N., & Penson, W. (2015). Expert views of peer-based interventions for prisoner health. *International Journal of Prisoner Health*, 11(2), 87–97. https://doi.org/10.1108/IJPH-10-2014-0039

Wright, N., Bleakley, A., Butt, C., Chadwick, O., Mahmood, K., Patel, K., et al. (2011). Peer health promotion in prisons: A systematic review. *International Journal of Prisoner Health*, 7(4), 37–51. https://doi.org/10.1108/17449201111256899

Other Areas
of Interest

14

DEFINITION

This chapter is composed of interesting interventions in areas other than those categorized in the main chapters. These did not result from a specific search of the literature, since clearly Other Areas of Interest is not a viable search term, but were noticed as the searches for other topics were conducted. They do however show the considerable breadth and scope of the peer intervention methodology.

REVIEWS OF EVIDENCE

There were five reviews of topics beyond the main categorizations. Three of these were reviews of peer intervention in social isolation and will be discussed first. Laermans et al. (2023) discussed friendly visiting by a volunteer for reducing loneliness or social isolation in older adults. A befriending intervention whereby older persons are matched with someone who visits them face-to-face on a regular basis seems promising but is it effective? The effects on feelings of loneliness, social isolation and wellbeing in older adults (≥60 years of age) were investigated. Six electronic databases were searched up until 2021. Experimental and observational studies were included that quantitatively measured the effect of intervention, compared to no friendly visiting, on at least one of the outcomes. Data were extracted for short-term, intermediate-term and long-term. Nine RCTs and four non-RCTs, conducted primarily in the United States and involving a total of 470 older adults (ages 72–83 years), were included. Programs lasted 6–12 weeks, and mostly involved weekly visits by undergraduate students to community-dwelling older adults. Due to the very low-certainty evidence, it was not clear whether visiting was effective, either in the short or long term.

Older people were also the focus of research by Meehan et al. (2023). Loneliness and social isolation were being redefined as public health issues, being associated with significant health risks, particularly in older people. A total of 52 articles from 30 countries met the inclusion criteria, including 33 observational studies, primarily cross-sectional (88%) and 19 interventions, mostly (89%) pre-post evaluations. The majority of included articles measured loneliness only ($n = 34$, 65%), while 11 measured both loneliness and social isolation (21%). To measure these outcomes, validated scales were frequently used. Neighborhood safety, access to public third places and cultural practices were investigated in relation to loneliness. Community-based interventions were either educational or enlisted volunteers to foster connections. Mahon (2024) focused on loneliness and social isolation in adults and young people. Loneliness and social isolation were risk factors for morbidity and mortality and a growing health concern. Five databases were searched for peer-reviewed literature published till 2023. The search yielded 2,402 articles of which 12 met the inclusion criteria. Emerging areas of interest included the use of technology to deliver interventions and the use of technology to facilitate peer support implementation with populations difficult to reach. There are several other reviews of loneliness and social isolation. This term could be searched for.

Turning to other topics, Freestone et al. (2022) offered a scoping review of peer interventions for gay and bisexual men who have sex with men. Five electronic databases were searched and 38 studies included. These covered peer counseling [$n = 6$], groupwork programs [$n = 15$], peer navigation [$n = 7$] and peer education [$n = 10$]. Most addressed HIV [$n = 32$]. Across intervention modalities, evaluations demonstrated compelling evidence of significant effect.

An interesting systematic review and meta-analysis of community-based interventions for stillbirths in sub-Saharan Africa was offered by Gwacham-Anisiobi et al. (2024). Sub-Saharan Africa alone contributed 42% of global stillbirths in 2019. The objective was to examine the effect of community-based interventions on stillbirth in this area. Eight databases were searched plus grey literature from 2000 to 2023. The study outcome was odds of stillbirth in intervention versus control communities. Of the 4,223 records identified, 17 studies from 15 countries were eligible for inclusion. The odds of stillbirth did not vary significantly between community-based intervention and control groups [Odds Ratio (OR) 0.96, $n = 63,884$]. However, analysis of four (out of five) studies that included both community and health facility components found that in comparison with community-only interventions, this combination strategy significantly reduced the odds of stillbirth by

17% (OR 0.83, $n = 244,868$). This combination seemed necessary to have a substantial effect.

SINGLE STUDIES

Number of Single Studies

There were nine single studies, but of course these were not searched for.

Exemplar Single Studies Developed Context

Hu et al. (2014) evaluated the effects of a sun-safe peer education program in China. A cluster random control intervention involved two primary schools, two grades in each school; three classes in each grade were randomly designated as intervention ($n = 304$) and control ($n = 305$). Thirty-six students were selected as peer educators and trained for one month. Peer education then took place for one month. Changes in sun-safe knowledge, attitude and behavior were conducted before intervention and at months 0, 1 and 6. After the intervention, sun-safe knowledge remarkably improved, compared to baseline survey ($p < 0.001$) and it sustained at this high level, while control group students' scores did not change ($p = 0.410$).

The effectiveness of a short educational intervention delivered by professional rugby union players in youth sport to reduce use of homophobic language was studied by Denison et al. (2023). In a cluster randomized controlled trial, 13 Australian youth rugby teams from nine clubs ($N = 167$, ages 16–20 years) were randomized to intervention or control groups. Professional rugby players delivered the intervention in-person. Frequency of homophobic language use was measured two weeks before and two weeks after the intervention. At baseline, 49% of participants self-reported using homophobic language in the past two weeks and 73% reported teammates using homophobic language. However, the intervention did not significantly reduce homophobic language. Kia et al. (2023) used virtual, semi-structured interviews with 35 transgender individuals in two Canadian cities who indicated having experiences of seeking, receiving and/or providing peer support. Broadly, transgender peers could enhance gender-affirming care by (1) validating a growing diversity of embodiments and experiences in healthcare decision-making, (2) nurturing and diversifying relevant networks of safety, community support and advocacy outside formal systems of care, and (3) strengthening possibilities for resisting and transforming existing healthcare systems.

Exemplar Single Studies Developing Context

Tinago et al. (2023) tested the effectiveness of a community-based peer support intervention to mitigate social isolation and the stigma of adolescent motherhood in Zimbabwe. Community health workers ($n = 12$) and peer educators ($n = 12$) were recruited and trained on co-facilitating peer support groups. Adolescent mothers aged 15–18 years from two low-income, high-density communities were recruited. The intervention arm ($n = 104$) participated in the peer support groups (control arm $n = 79$). Peer support groups (12 groups with 6–12 participants in each) met in-person twice a month and completed 12 sessions addressing participant-identified topics such as income generation and depression. WhatsApp Messenger was used for training and implementation support. The intervention arm reported lower depressive symptoms and mental disorder and higher overall, family, friends and significant-other support, compared to control. The intervention arm felt more engaged with peers, knew who and where to turn to for help, and had coping, parenting and communication strategies to manage life challenges.

Somewhat similarly, Kåks et al. (2024) evaluated a social innovation for community-based peer support for immigrant mothers in Sweden. The objective was to support expectant women and mothers of young children in immigrant communities to access public services that would benefit maternal and child health. Semi-structured interviews ($n = 19$) were conducted with peer supporters, client mothers and key stakeholders. The five peer supporters had 1,294 contacts with client mothers, of which 507 were first-time contacts. The dose of the intervention was tailored to individual needs. Peer supporters tended to prioritize linking clients to other services over the educational components of the intervention, sometimes doing more than what was originally planned. Implementation strategies used included building trust, using multiple outreach venues, using internal support structures and providing practical assistance. The personal connection between peer supporters and clients was highly valued, and the building of relationships enabled them to address sensitive topics.

Moshki et al. (2017) used peer education in an RCT in Iran for adopting preventive behaviors against head lice infestation in female elementary school students. This condition is more prevalent in populous and deprived communities with poor personal hygiene. A total of 179 female fifth-grade students were selected and randomly allocated to control and intervention groups. A questionnaire was designed and administered to collect baseline information. The educational program consisted of three sessions, held by peers for the intervention group. The questionnaire was re-administered one month after the intervention. Initially, the two groups had no significant differences. After the intervention, however, the mean scores of all parameters significantly improved in the intervention group.

SPECIFIC PROGRAM

Effectiveness

Avci et al. (2023) studied the effect of a peer education model on reducing smartphone addiction in adolescents, the group at highest risk of addiction and exacerbated by the covid pandemic. The study was a pre-test–post-test control group design, carried out with 622 high school students in Turkey. In the first stage, the peer educator education program on smartphone addiction in adolescents was implemented. In the second stage, the peer education program was implemented and monitored. While there was no significant difference between the intervention and control groups in terms of the mean scores they obtained from the Smartphone Addiction Scale (SAS) at the pre-test ($p > 0.05$), the difference between them was statistically significant at the post-test ($p < 0.001$).

Implementation

The study was carried out in two stages. The first stage included the implementation of the training program for peer educators on smartphone addiction in adolescents, and the second stage included the implementation and monitoring of the peer education program.

First stage: Implementation of the peer educator education program

The aim of the program was to educate peer educators who would provide information about smartphone addiction to adolescents. First, relevant sample education programs and education model guides were examined by the researchers. Then, the training program, including peer education, effective communication skills, smartphone addiction and effective presentation skills, was prepared.

The peer educator training program was announced by hanging posters on the boards of the intervention school. A total of 24 students, one girl and one boy from each classroom, were selected from among the students who volunteered. The opinions of the class counselor and teachers about the extent to which students met the National Peer Counselors Association criteria (communication skills, helpfulness, responsibility, leadership, reliability, honesty and sensitivity) were taken into account. Then, a parent permission request was sent to the parents of the students selected, which informed them about the study and asked them to allow their children to participate in the study. Their consent was obtained.

Before the program was started, interviews were held with the peer educator candidates. In this interview, the Personal Information Form (PIF) and the SAS were administered to the prospective peer educators as a pre-test. Then, the schedule for implementation was planned. It was carried out by two researchers. The program consisted of six sessions, each 90 minutes, and was completed in three weeks with two sessions per week. The education sessions were supported by visual and written materials and were carried out in the form of interactive education. Reinforcers and psychodramas were utilized to encourage the prospective peer educators to continue participating in the group, to act appropriately and to communicate effectively with each other.

Below is the brief information about the content of the six sessions:

a. *First session*: mutual acquaintance between peer educators, developing a sense of trust, structuring the group process, determining the group rules and name, signing the group agreement and introducing the program and its general objectives;

b. *Second session*: explaining the concept of peer education, making students realize the importance of peer education practices and discussing the tasks and responsibilities of peer educators. In addition, this week, a trip activity was held in order to improve the communication between the participants and to motivate them.

c. *Third session*: explaining the concept of communication, basic features of communication and effective communication skills; discussing the importance of effective communication skills and making them notice their own communication skills.

d. *Fourth session*: explaining the concept of addiction; types of addiction; smartphone addiction; the prevalence, causes and consequences of smartphone addiction and the fight against smartphone addiction.

e. *Fifth session*: explanation of education methods and techniques and discussion of effective presentation skills.

f. *Sixth session*: evaluation of the program, sharing the gains and skills acquired, rehearsing the presentation and sharing feelings and thoughts about ending the sessions.

In order to evaluate effectiveness, the peer educators were interviewed again two weeks after the program. In this interview, the SAS was administered as a post-test. In addition, the peer education process was briefly explained again, and the preparations were evaluated. Then, the students who attended all of the sessions were given peer educator certificates.

When the effectiveness of the implemented program was evaluated, the mean SAS score of students was 30.16 before the program and 15.58 after the program, and the difference was statistically significant ($p < 0.001$).

Second stage: Implementation and monitoring of the peer education program

Before the program was started, the students in the intervention and control groups were informed about the study, and an informed consent form indicating that they volunteered to participate in the study was sent to their parents and their consent was obtained.

' Two weeks before implementation, the PIF and the SAS were administered as a pre-test to the intervention and control groups by the researchers. The participants in the control group did not undergo any interventions. Then, in order for the program to be implemented for two hours, planning took into account the curriculum of all classes, and the peer education program was carried out with the students in the intervention group. First, peer educators informed other students in their classes about the content and purpose of the peer education program. Afterward, a visual presentation was given on smartphone addiction, and a short film about phone addiction displayed. After the education, the peer educators obtained the opinions of the peers about the program, and their questions were answered.

In addition, for two weeks, peer educators continued to share their knowledge about smartphone addiction with their friends in the classroom or in social environments. During implementation, peer educators were provided with counseling and support services, when necessary, by the researchers. Two weeks after the completion of the peer education program, the SAS was administered to the intervention and control groups as a post-test.

REFERENCES

Avci, D., Gündoğdu, N. A., Dönmez, R. H., & Avci, F. E. (2023). Students as teachers: Effect of the peer education model on reducing smartphone addiction in adolescents. *Health Education Research*, *38*(2), 107–118. https://doi.org/10.1093/her/cyac042

Denison, E., Faulkner, N., O'Brien, K. S., Jeanes, R., & Canning, M. (2023). Effectiveness of an educational intervention targeting homophobic language use by young male athletes: A cluster randomised controlled trial. *British Journal of Sports Medicine*, *57*(9), 515–520. https://doi.org/10.1136/bjsports-2022-105916

Freestone, J., Siefried, K. J., Prestage, G., Hammoud, M., Molyneux, A., & Bourne, A. (2022). Individual level peer interventions for gay and bisexual men who have sex with men between 2000 and 2020: A scoping review. *PLoS ONE*, *17*(7), e0270649. https://doi.org/10.1371/journal.pone.0270649

Gwacham-Anisiobi, U., Boo, Y. Y., Oladimeji, A., Kurinczuk, J. J., Roberts, N., & Opondo, C., et al. (2024). Effects of community-based interventions for stillbirths in sub-saharan Africa: A systematic review and meta-analysis. *eClinicalMedicine*, *67*, 102386. https://doi.org/10.1016/j.eclinm.2023.102386

Hu, P., Han, L. L., Sharma, M., Zeng, H., Zhang, Y., & Hui, L., et al. (2014). Evaluation of cognitive and behavioral effects of peer education model-based intervention to sun safe in children. *Iranian Journal of Public Health*, *43*(3), 300–309.

Kåks, P., Stansert, K. L., Målqvist, M., Bergström, A., & Herzig, vS. (2024). Implementing A social innovation for community-based peer support for immigrant mothers in Sweden: A mixed-methods process evaluation. *Frontiers in Public Health*, *11*, 1332738. https://doi.org/10.3389/fpubh.2023.1332738

Kia, H., Kenney, K. A., Abramovich, A., Ferlatte, O., MacKinnon, K. R., & Knight, R. (2023). "Nowhere else to be found": Drawing on peer support experiences among transgender and gender-diverse people to substantiate community-driven gender-affirming care. *Social Science & Medicine*, *339*, 116406. https://doi.org/10.1016/j.socscimed.2023.116406

Laermans, J., Scheers, H., Vandekerckhove, P., & De Buck, E. (2023). Friendly Visiting by a volunteer for reducing loneliness or social isolation in older adults: A systematic review. *Campbell Systematic Reviews*, *19*(4), e1359. https://doi.org/10.1002/cl2.1359

Mahon, D. (2024). Scoping review of peer support for adults and young people experiencing loneliness and social isolation. *Mental Health and Social Inclusion*. https://doi.org/10.1108/MHSI-11-2023-0129

Meehan, D. E., Grunseit, A., Condie, J., HaGani, N., & Merom, D. (2023). Social-ecological factors influencing loneliness and social isolation in older people: A scoping review. *BMC Geriatrics*, *23*(1), Article number 726. https://doi.org/10.1186/s12877-023-04418-8

Moshki, M., Zamani-Alavijeh, F., & Mojadam, M. (2017). Efficacy of peer education for adopting preventive behaviors against head lice infestation in female elementary school students: A randomised controlled trial. *PLoS ONE*, *12*(1), e0169361. https://doi.org/10.1371/journal.pone.0169361

Tinago, C. B., Frongillo, E. A., Warren, A. M., Chitiyo, V., Jackson, T. N., Cifarelli, A. K., et al. (2023). Testing the effectiveness of a community-based peer support intervention to mitigate social isolation and stigma of adolescent motherhood in Zimbabwe. *Maternal and Child Health Journal*, *8*(4), 657–666. https://doi.org/10.1007/s10995-023-03821-2

Implementation 15

This chapter was developed from consideration of the (relatively scarce) literature on core competencies and tasks required for successful implementation of peer interventions (Kotera et al., 2023; Larimer et al., 2022; Lekka et al., 2015; Mark et al., 2019; McCrary et al., 2022) and careful inspection of the specific programs outlining implementation in each chapter of this book. All of these were set in the context of a particular health problem or wellbeing outcome, so merging them and developing implementation guidelines for *all* health and wellbeing areas required considerable generalization. Eighteen different variables were finally identified, displayed in Table 15.1. When planning a peer intervention, it is suggested that all 18 be carefully considered.

TABLE 15.1 Variables in ensuring effective peer interventions

	VARIABLE
1	Cultural Context
2	Recruiting Organizations
3	Pilot Consultations
4	Peer Helper Role
5	Mode of Delivery
6	Peer Helper Recruitment
7	Peer Helper Training
8	Assessment of Training Effects
9	Equipment including Digital Technology
10	Matching and First Contact
11	Frequency and Duration
12	Activity
13	Contract
14	Record-keeping and Monitoring
15	Support for Peer Helpers
16	Implementation Fidelity
17	Acknowledgement and Remuneration
18	Retention and Longer-Term Planning

DOI: 10.1201/9781003438366-15

This table is also available as a Word download in Appendix 2 Online Only (https://www.routledge.com/9781032572109) so readers may customize it to their purposes.

CULTURAL CONTEXT

Consideration has to be given to the social, cultural, political and organizational context in which peer intervention is to be situated. Firstly, consider the cultural context within the medical profession and para-profession. Is the country developed enough for there to be adequate staffing and resources for medical staff to be able to help with the project? Do they have time and are they flexible enough? Do some of them have negative attitudes to peer intervention, which might sabotage the project? If there are not enough medical staff to help, consideration has to be given to community organizations and charities who might be willing to help run the project.

Secondly, consider the cultural context within the likely participants. Are there traditional beliefs and practices, myths and superstitions, which might militate against a successful project? Some of these will be relatively obvious (e.g., a belief that breast milk is insufficient to nourish babies), while others may be more tangential (e.g., a belief that training should be highly didactic and teacher-centered). Nonetheless, the research shows that peer support has a significantly greater effect on low- or middle-income countries in some areas, e.g., reducing the risk of not breast feeding at all by 30% compared to 7% in high-income countries. Similarly, the risk of non-exclusive breast feeding decreased significantly more in low- or middle-income countries.

Thirdly, consider the social context. Are there societal divisions which inhibit one group of people communicating with another group? Are there multiple languages in play which further inhibit such communication?

Finally, consider the political context. If local or central government is resistant to the idea of peer intervention (perhaps because they are wedded to a model more prevalent in wealthy Western countries), there may well be difficulties.

RECRUITING ORGANIZATIONS

Involving local organizations will be important to developing a successful project, especially in terms of sustainability when the project initiators pull out. Schools and colleges are an obvious example of organizations, which could be key to successful implementation, but they would need to actively buy into the project, and not just at management or administrator level. Helping schools and colleges meet national policy requirements would be a strong motivator. The intervention could help schools meet relevant indicators, particularly around enhancing students' confidence and sense of responsibility and addressing stigmatizing attitudes. Project leaders should actively seek a range of different types of organizations with whom to partner.

PILOT CONSULTATIONS

Before starting a project, informal consultations are necessary with key stakeholders, who include medical staff and local organizations, but importantly also potential participants from the target group under consideration, as a kind of needs assessment. These groups will have ideas about what kind of intervention is likely to be most acceptable to the participants (they may of course all have different ideas) and be able to advise about the structure of the intervention. Initial consultations with young people are particularly required. These may take the form of individual interviews or focus group meetings, located in an organization like a school or college, or outside in a community organization. The number of participants might vary between six and 36. Young people often express a desire for relatable experiential information and suggest that the use of humor and interactive components would enhance training and online content. Discussion is likely to include challenges associated with treatment uptake, key issues facing people beyond the clinic, modes of communication and gender norms, and accessibility of technology.

PEER HELPER ROLE

Peer interveners work under a variety of titles, which do not clearly define their duties. Are they peer educators, peer counselors or peer supporters? Or one of the other terms variously used: peer mentors, peer navigators, peer coaches and so on? In principle, the role of peer educator, counselors and supporters can be differentiated. Peer educators tend to operate in groups and focus on imparting knowledge (albeit with a hope that this will influence later behavior). Peer counselors are more likely to work on a one-to-one basis, although they can also work in groups (c.f., Alcoholics Anonymous), and tend to focus on social aspects and behavioral intentions in terms of steps toward recovery. Peer supporters are even more likely to work on a one-to-one basis, given that the support they offer is highly individualized and more focused on the emotional components, and are likely to set goals for behavioral and physiological improvement.

However, in many cases, these roles become blurred in practice. Peers may start off as educators then become more engaged in the social and emotional aspects and transition into peer counselors. Peer counselors may develop a stronger affinity to individualized work and transition into peer supporters. The training provided should in any case seek to address all three types of roles to a greater or lesser extent, since peer interveners are likely to find they encounter situations which are otherwise outside their comfort zone. Sequenced training over time could build from one to the other role. Of course, peer helper personal preferences will suggest what kind of role they are suited for, but these preferences may change over time as a product of experience. Will peer interveners be comfortable working with participants older than they are, or will this need to be learned? In any event, a clear title for the peer interveners will be needed. This is a question best put to participants in a pilot consultation meeting.

MODE OF DELIVERY

First thoughts are likely to suggest face-to-face meetings, but these may be difficult if the participants are very scattered and local peer interveners cannot be identified. Are face-to-face meetings to be individual or group or a mixture of the two? Digital communication may be a useful way of at least issuing reminders (perhaps via text messaging) to participants about face-to-face meetings and working toward their goals, but here limited access to devices and to the internet may prove a barrier. Some peer interventions are completely online (known as TeleHealth), but the access issue is even more prominent in this case. It is of course possible to have group sessions online via video conferencing, but this requires reliable bandwidth. A project may have a website containing information, which participants can visit whenever they do have internet access.

PEER HELPER RECRUITMENT

There are very different views on how peer helpers should be recruited. Some projects rely on recommendations from professionals or organizations who know the participants, but a more radical way is to choose peer interveners on the basis of a vote count from their peer group. Other projects have an open invitation, which is widely advertised.

As an example of the first way, discussions with class teachers led to the researchers selecting four excellent, prestigious and well-communicated students (two boys and two girls) who were class committee members and actively participated in extracurricular activities. Alternatively, potential peer leaders were identified through recommendations from health professionals and were mostly female and university educated. Alternatively, the opinions of the class counselor and teachers about the extent to which students met the National Peer Counselors Association criteria (communication skills, helpfulness, responsibility, leadership, reliability, honesty and sensitivity) were taken into account. All this highlights the problem that nominations from professionals may be weak at identifying peers who could become powerful interveners.

As an example of the second way, all students were asked to nominate the most influential and compassionate students in their grade group. Those who received the most nominations were invited to become peer educators. Elsewhere, all students were asked to complete a peer nomination questionnaire. Questions included:

1. Who do you respect in your year at your school?
2. Who are good leaders in sports or other group activities in your year?
3. Who do you look up to in your year?
4. With whom in your year would you feel comfortable to talk about something personal or sensitive?
5. Who in your year is good at encouraging and persuading others to do things?
6. Whose opinion do you trust and value most in your year?
7. Who in your year is confident at talking to people outside their friendship group?

Alternatively, each of the village local council chairpersons organized a meeting with women in their respective villages. At these meetings, the study team explained to the women what the study was about and the need to identify one of their number to be trained as peer counselor for breastfeeding. The women proposed two to three candidates who were then interviewed by the study team. To be selected, a woman had to be aged between 18 and 45 years and to be resident in the area with no plans of leaving the area within two years. She had to have a good reputation in the community. Further, she had to be literate and numerate in the local language, willing to participate in the study including a one-week training and to undertake home visits in order to help women breastfeed their babies.

As an example of the third way, participants were recruited from paid advertisements placed on Google and Facebook and also disseminated through various American Cancer Society webpages, the SmokefreeTXT sign-up webpage, Facebook webpages dedicated to smoking cessation, solicitation of facilitators of the Freshstart® group-based cessation support program, online notices on webpages and posts to online smoking cessation forums. All advertisements directed participants to the study website, which included study details and a screening survey.

A key issue is whether peer helpers are to have a history of recovery themselves from the problem in question. Generally, the research evidence suggests that if they do, this is likely to make their intervention more powerful.

PEER HELPER TRAINING

The first step in designing an effective training program is to examine other relevant programs in your area of practice, particularly their practical manuals. These may be good, bad or indifferent, but will at least give some idea of the parameters of the field. Secondly, consider you own views about pedagogy (if you are not a teacher, you might not have any). Perhaps you are in a country where the dominant pedagogy in practice (whatever policy documents say) is highly didactic and teacher-centered. While this may be effective to an extent in peer education, it will be of little use for peer counseling and peer support, where individual person-centered communication skills are much more important. In some programs, professional trainers were used to train peer supporters to increase intervention efficacy and credibility and reduce the burden on schools. However, other programs used a train-the-trainer model in which experienced peers taught other inexperienced volunteers the various roles required. For example, the AA program encourages individuals who are in recovery to invite newcomers to share their stories and adopt a mentoring role.

Example of a Training Program

The program consisted of six sessions, each 90 minutes, and was completed in three weeks with two sessions per week. Sessions were supported by visual and written materials and constituted interactive education. Reinforcers and psychodramas were utilized to encourage the prospective peer educators to communicate effectively with each other.

a. *First session*: mutual acquaintance between peer educators, developing a sense of trust, structuring the group process, determining the group rules and name, signing the group agreement and introducing the program and its general objectives;

b. *Second session*: explaining the concept of peer education, making students realize the importance of peer education practices and discussing the tasks and responsibilities of peer educators. In addition, a trip activity was held in order to improve the communication between the participants and to motivate them.

c. *Third session*: explaining the concept of communication, basic features of communication and effective communication skills; discussing the importance of effective communication skills and helping them notice their own communication skills.

d. *Fourth session*: explaining the concept of addiction; types of addiction; smartphone addiction; the prevalence, causes and consequences of smartphone addiction and the fight against smartphone addiction.

e. *Fifth session*: explanation of education methods and techniques and discussion of effective presentation skills.

f. *Sixth session*: evaluation of the program, sharing the gains and skills acquired, rehearsing the presentation and sharing feelings and thoughts about ending the sessions.

Didactic Teacher-Centered Models of Instruction

Didactic teacher-centered training courses could focus on up-to-date information about community resources and services. Training could include six modules with an accompanying slide deck that took two hours to complete, with a quiz at the end of each module. Workshops could consist of lecture presentations, written materials, videotapes and interactive exercises. Content could include key issues facing this population, including stigma, disclosure, socioeconomic issues and gender-based violence. The training could also include maintaining confidentiality and boundaries of providing peer support.

Learner-Centered Communication Skills Models of Instruction

Relationship building skills are key to person-centered interaction. This includes the use of respectful, person-centered, recovery-oriented language in written and verbal interactions with peers, family members, community members and others, the use of active listening skills, clarifying client understanding of information, conveying the client's point of view when working with colleagues, documenting information as required by program policies and procedures, following laws and rules concerning confidentiality, and respecting others' right to privacy.

Lived experiences of recovery should be shared. Helpers are encouraged to draw on their own experiences as parents, friends, siblings or caregivers. They relate personal recovery stories and, with permission, the recovery stories of others, to inspire hope, discuss ongoing personal efforts to enhance health, wellness and recovery, recognizing when to share experiences and when to listen, describe personal recovery practices and help peers discover recovery practices that work for them.

Peer intervention should be personalized. It requires an understanding of personal values and cultures and how these may contribute to biases, judgments and beliefs, and an appreciation of and respect for the cultural and spiritual beliefs and practices of peers and their families. Helpers learn to recognize and respond to the complexities and uniqueness of each peers' process of recovery and tailor services and support to meet the preferences and unique needs of peers and their families.

Goal setting involves open-ended and closed-ended questions and paraphrasing and using problem solving or definition of the main problem. Peers should be assisted and supported to set goals and dream about future possibilities, propose strategies to help accomplish tasks or goals, and use decision-making strategies when choosing services and support.

Peer helpers also assist peers in investigating, selecting and using needed and desired resources and services, accompanying peers to community activities and appointments when requested, and participating in community activities with peers when requested. They also work together with other colleagues to enhance the provision of services, assertively engage providers from other services to meet the needs of peers, coordinate efforts with health care providers, coordinate efforts with peers' family members and other natural supports, partner with community members and organizations to strengthen opportunities for peers, and strive to resolve relationship conflicts with peers and others in their support network.

Goals of Instruction

During training, peer educators should be instructed on how to be sensitive, open-minded, good listeners and how to communicate their ideas and feelings in a positive and non-judgmental way, as well as how to project a positive attitude and how to recognize and respond to problems among friends. This equips them with the knowledge, skills and confidence required for the role; builds motivation and enthusiasm for the role; generates trust and rapport within the group; builds knowledge and skills; improves understanding of risks and consequences; builds self-esteem and self-efficacy; reinforces social support for healthy norms; and boosts intrinsic motivation and autonomy. Peer-led facilitation allows young people to express themselves freely, develop a sense of self-worth and interact more. The nature of mobile technology also allowed participants to build friendships beyond their geographic area and interact with their peers in real time.

Time and Duration

The frequency and duration of training sessions varied enormously. For example, peer support groups (e.g., 12 groups with 6–12 participants in each) met in-person twice a month and completed 12 sessions, addressing participant-identified topics. Others were given two days of training, six days of training, 12 hours of training, 40-hour intensive training, a 60-minute training session every day for five days, ten educational sessions of 50–55 minutes or several weeks of training. Generally, it will be more effective if training sessions are spaced to allow some absorption and reflection in between.

Pedagogical Methods

Close consideration should be given to the most effective format for training activities. Activities should prioritize smaller group work and fewer topics should be covered, but in more depth (with remaining topics moved to the follow-up sessions). Information and skills training should be integrated across days, rather than allocated one day each.

Different methods, including lectures, film presentations, group discussions, question and answer sessions and role playing, can be used. Training can include knowledge contests and self-made poster exhibitions (knowledge quiz software was provided, as were group discussion cases and analysis results, role-playing scripts and related pubertal health education slides). In another program, the modules covered study details, guidance rooted in motivational interviewing techniques regarding how to advise mentees, and a tutorial about the study's web-based text-messaging platform. In yet another, peer-elected leaders moderated monthly meetings involving role-play, brainstorming and activities. Nine behavior change techniques were identified, with the most used being information about health consequences and social and emotional consequences, demonstration of behavior, behavioral practice/rehearsal and instructions on how to perform the behavior.

Peer helpers were trained on facilitation skills and techniques such as active listening, empathetic encouragement, non-judgmental communication, asking open-ended questions, validation and problem solving. The facilitators were briefed on the technological platform, including trouble shooting and referral processes. The final part involved scenario-based thinking, where participants were given difficult issues to engage with and resolve that might occur in the groups, such as conflict between participants. In another program, the focus was patient centered: listening, reflecting and avoiding unsolicited advice.

In another program, participants practiced approaches for communicating with and supporting partners' needs using individual, dyadic and group reflective exercises, discussion and shared problem solving, interactive skill sessions and writing exercises. They learned through (a) peer-to-peer sharing, (b) problem solving and brainstorming, and (c) leadership and experiential activities. Participatory learning was used, encouraging participants to share their opinions, generate innovative ideas, make informed decisions, evaluate personal experiences, make training enjoyable and apply principles learned to everyday life. In yet another project, a horseshoe seating arrangement conveyed a sense of visual connectedness and 'equality of status' among learners. Peers completed problem-solving exercises as a large group and in dyads, typically using case scenarios and prepared exercises. These varied from simple exercises to role-playing to opportunities to create new training content. The brainstorming/problem-posing exercises, in contrast, were used to create options for resolving hypothetical and real-life problems.

Other methods included following a cast of characters and a storyline that was sustained throughout the sessions, using visual cartoon characters. Yet another comprised six sessions based on audio-taped stories told by teenagers (two boys and two girls), who described their life events, sharing their feelings and opinions, containing cartoons that described the adventures of two young detectives who tried to protect children from problems.

ASSESSMENT OF TRAINING EFFECTS

Once initial training has been completed, there needs to be some assessment of whether it was effective before peer helpers are unleashed on unsuspecting clients. Assessment not only needs to cover knowledge, but also attitudes, behavioral intentions and even practice in a simulated scenario. Knowledge can be assessed by a test with both open-ended and closed questions, as well as assessing attitudes and beliefs. This could be done at pre-test to reveal problems, which could then be addressed in the subsequent training. Some criteria need to be established to determine adequate performance on this assessment. If the participant does not score highly enough, they may need to be eliminated from the helper pool. Some areas of performance may be seen as more crucial than others, so performance is weighted accordingly. Regarding simulated scenarios, which are very useful for assessing person-centered communication skills, peer counselors can be involved in a minimum of two videotaped practice role-playing contacts. After this, they could attend two one-hour sessions where two members of the research team provide assessment of each videotaped intervention. Both tapes could have been previously coded by the researchers. Assessment of specific behaviors such as use of open-ended questions can be done. If a manual is provided, key competences listed in the manual can be assessed.

For example, in one project, potential peer helpers completed a 15 to 20-minute practice phone counseling conversation via telephone with a research team member one week after the conclusion of their training. All practice conversations were recorded, and peers received immediate verbal feedback from the research team member. The recordings were coded. Global ratings included two components: one to capture counselor empathy (i.e., the extent to which the interviewer understood and/or made an effort to grasp the partner's perspective) and the second for spirit (i.e., the overall competence of the interviewer in using evocation, collaboration and autonomy), each rated from 1 to 5, with higher scores indicating higher success. The second domain, behavioral counts, tallied four specific behaviors: (1) reflection to question ratio; (2) percent open-ended questions; (3) percent complex questions; and (4) percentage adherent or non-adherent statements.

EQUIPMENT INCLUDING DIGITAL TECHNOLOGY

Even for exclusively face-to-face projects, some kind of equipment will be needed, usually a manual which covers they key behaviors needed to be shown by peer helpers during the intervention. This manual may need to be produced in several different languages (and of course the peer helpers need to be literate). Examples are:

- Peer supporter handbook, PATA 2017: https://teampata.org/portfolio/2829/
- Community health worker and peer supporter toolkit, PATA 2017: https://teampata.org/portfolio/3548/
- Good practice guide for adolescent HIV programming, International HIV/AIDS Alliance and READY +, 2017: https://www.aidsalliance.org/resources/922-goodpractice-guide-adolescent-hiv-programming
- Case study on Africaid-Zvandiri CATS model, International HIV/AIDS Alliance 2018: https://www.youtube.com/watch?v=2h82W4OYx4A and https://teampata.org/wp-content/uploads/2018/12/web_Y-clinic-leaflet-ENG-2018_UPDATED.pdf
- Peer leader manual published by the International Diabetes Federation: https://idf.org/media/uploads/2023/05/attachments-35.pdf
- The National Heart, Lung, and Blood Institute booklet: With Every Heartbeat Is Life: A Community Health Worker's Manual for African Americans. https://www.nhlbi.nih.gov/education/heart-truth/CHW/WEHL
- La Leche South Africa breastfeeding: https://www.lllsa.org/product-page/breastfeeding-peer-counsellor-online-training-program
- WHO breastfeeding: https://iris.who.int/bitstream/handle/10665/63428/WHO_CDR_93.4-eng.pdf?sequence=1
- Peer Connect is a program at the University of North Carolina at Chapel Hill's LIVESTRONG Survivorship Center of Excellence (http://carolinawell.org/connecting.do)
- Service provider guidance for working with young people living with HIV, Y + 2018: https://books.google.co.uk/books?hl=en&lr=&id=UI5FEAAAQBAJ&oi=fnd&pg=PR5&dq=Service+provider+guidance+for+working+with+young+people+living+with+HIV,+Y+%2B+2018:&ots=pQVzo3UQ-D&sig=eHTajAVFoMe8lixLfyz1Ac8GyY0#v=onepage&q&f=false

In addition, simple illustrated brochures can be distributed to the clients to explain the harmful effects of various unwanted behaviors, the peer pressure effect and how to say no and avoid engaging in any unhealthy behaviors.

Other interventions can be either blended (a combination of digital and face-to-face) or exclusively digital. In either case, accessibility of devices and to the internet are highly relevant, and this may not be the case in poorer communities. Projects may need to give devices (usually mobile phones with contracts) to peer helpers and their clients, if funding can be found for such expense. For example, in one project, all participants received a new feature phone that had

SMS functionality (i.e., not a smart phone) and a registered SIM card to use during the intervention. Flickswitch© was the software used to control SIM cards, to distribute and top-up text messages airtime. Group SMS format was made possible with ZygoHubs© and BulkSMS© technology. Again, messages can be sent in several languages. Some of these messages can be automated (e.g., reminders to do necessary tasks), while others will be personalized to the client.

There may be a project website which has information, and this can reduce the burden of remembering all the required knowledge by peer helpers. Peer helpers can use this themselves for revision of knowledge and also direct clients to the relevant section of the website. It can include brief study guides, audio/video presentations that support self-directed learning and access to other educational resources, including electronic versions of the manual. Ideally, groups of clients should give opinions on draft website content.

Applications for transmitting messages will vary by country and region and may be locally developed, although Facebook, Instagram, WhatsApp and Snapchat are widely used. Candidate social media platforms need to be reviewed for user demographics, functionality, appeal and regulatory information. Platforms need the following priorities for functionality: appeal to young people; provide options to post web links, images and/or text; provide an option to create private, invite-only groups; ease of viewing messages and message stability; potential for monitoring; and potential for interface with a website. Local examples include SmokefreeTXT (SFTXT), a nationwide text-messaging service provided by the National Cancer Institute in the USA. SFTXT provides 41 different behavior change techniques, including goal setting, problem solving, self-monitoring, feedback and social support. It delivers one to five automated messages per day for up to two weeks prior to a user-selected quit date and six weeks post-quit date.

Messages will vary over the course of the intervention. First, messages should be more conversational in tone, including conversation starters that prompt users to reply. Peer helpers could receive a message library, along with examples of follow-up prompts and probes that could be employed with each conversation starter. Helpers could edit automated messages to tailor them to each participant. Helpers could also send spontaneous (unscripted) messages at any time.

MATCHING AND FIRST CONTACT

Some thought needs to be given to matching peer helpers with clients. Ideally, all helpers will have somewhat recovered from the problem at hand. In some projects, gender may be a key factor. Age can also be an issue–while clients may speak more readily to someone of their own age, an older person might be wiser. Race can also be an issue—messages from someone of similar race tend to be more acted upon than other sorts. First contacts are important, and clients should be able to ask for a different peer helper if needed.

FREQUENCY AND DURATION

How often are contacts with peer helpers expected to be? How long will these contacts tend to be? How many weeks will the project last for? Most projects will set limits for these variables, but some tailor the dose of the intervention to individual needs. What happens when the project ends? Peer helpers might well need to work with a new set of clients, but some of the old clients may be very reluctant to let go. Care is needed to avoid helpers coming under unreasonable pressure.

ACTIVITY

While the first contact is important, the second and third contacts are likely to be less focused on social and introductory issues and more on the problem area at hand. For example, in prisons, the Toe-by-Toe program is run by prisoners, supervised and facilitated by prison staff via monthly meetings. Participants are placed in support groups of 8–15 peers who share experiences. These support groups can be virtually enabled through a digital platform, where participants discuss—peer-to-peer, anytime, anywhere via text message—a range of issues pertinent to their needs.

CONTRACT

Peer helpers need to fully commit to a project and may be asked to sign a contract or code of conduct. Alternatively, to signal the responsibility inherent in the role, supporters might be asked to sign a 'charter' on completion of the training. This would reiterate role expectations and the study values. In prisons, listeners sign a contract that binds them to the same policies to which Samaritans working in the community adhere.

RECORD-KEEPING AND MONITORING

Many projects require peer helpers to keep a diary or log of client contacts, but care has to be taken not to make the burden of administration too great for the helpers. Entries can be fabricated or omitted and might not offer an accurate activity record. Record-keeping could include activity records, posters and activity photos. When and how often do project supervisors get to inspect the logs? In some projects study personnel monitored chat logs daily, and contacted helpers by email if they went more than a day without responding to participant questions. Supervisors can be tasked with intermittent engagement, monitoring for problematic behavior or conflict and identifying participants for onward referral. Supervision can come from non-peers or from peers. Other approaches might include mystery client visits, feedback boxes, client satisfaction surveys and scorecards. Such logs can of course also be used as one of the implementation fidelity or evaluation measures for the project, although analyzing them can take a long time. The supervisory team can also make records of their visits to peer helpers and any observed helping sessions. Minutes of monthly meetings can be recorded as well as the topics discussed at different meetings. With projects with a digital component, recordings of digital activity can be collected automatically (with the consent of helpers and clients).

SUPPORT FOR PEER HELPERS

Although being a peer helper is associated with longer-term positive effects on the deliverer, helpers will need support to deal with difficult cases, including those with considerable co-morbidity. Support needs to validate peer helpers' experiences and feelings, encourage the exploration and pursuit of community roles, convey hope about recovery, celebrate peers' efforts and accomplishments and provide concrete assistance to help peers accomplish tasks and goals. Members of the program can meet weekly to discuss problematic issues. For example, in prisons, community volunteers from supporting Samaritans branches attend listener meetings every two weeks to provide emotional support for listeners and to regulate the programs and address any emerging issues.

The supervisory team could visit each peer counsellor at least once every two weeks, checking logs for completeness. Any achievements and challenges could be discussed and ways forward agreed. Interesting experiences could be noted by the supervisory team for sharing with the whole group at a subsequent monthly meeting. Some supervisory teams observe each peer helper operating once per month. After the helper had finished helping, the supervisor could give her/him feedback on performance. The peer helpers could also be invited to monthly meetings with the supervisors. At these meetings, they could present and discuss reports about their activities, achievements and challenges.

Secondary peer helper follow-up training could be performed to consolidate relevant knowledge and how to cope with stress or negative events. There could be monthly 90-minute supplemental sessions for six months to reinforce skills, gain additional practice and problem-solve issues.

IMPLEMENTATION FIDELITY

Monitoring the range and quality of services provided by peer supporters is important, together with indicators that measure their meaningful integration and participation. Several studies used various methods to evaluate implementation fidelity, but few assessed adherence and competence through audio- and video-taping or direct observations. This needs considering for future projects. One review found programs with a sample size < 100, duration of intervention ≤ 6 months, baseline HbA1c < 8.5%, delivery by group and high frequency of contact all had statistically significant effects, and these were useful indicators of implementation integrity.

ACKNOWLEDGMENT AND REMUNERATION

It will be clear from the above considerations that peer helping can be a weighty and stressful task which consumes a great deal of time. Accordingly, peer helpers may well benefit from some form of remuneration if funds permit. On the other hand, offering remuneration too early in the recruitment process can result in the wrong kind of helpers being recruited. Think about the basis on which helpers might be paid–per client, per number of contacts or what? In one project, financial rewards ($100/day for each training day) were provided at training completion, while in another, the peer helpers were provided with a small allowance of about 10% of a teacher's monthly salary (around US$20 per month). However, half of the studies gave no payment to peer supporters.

Alternatively (or indeed as well as), helpers might receive some kind of certificate upon completion of their training, with a further certificate to come at the end of the project. Formal recognition could be provided by a local university or other prestigious organization. For example, helpers were given the opportunity to bank time spent on the study towards attainment of a Saltire Award (Scottish Volunteer Award scheme), on a week-to-week basis, commitment was rewarded by a 'Supporter of the Week' prize, participants received a $25 gift card for completing the follow-up and an additional $25 for sending by email a photograph of their salivary test results, helpers received $50 for completing the training, $150 for mentoring ($200 for accepting four mentees) and entry into a $1,000 draw. In prisons, employment is often categorized in bands, and each band is associated with different levels of privilege (i.e., extra and improved visits, access to in-cell television and the opportunity to wear one's own clothes). Peer helpers operate within the 'red band' and have the highest level of privileges.

RETENTION AND LONGER-TERM PLANNING

Starting the project is one thing, but planning for sustainability is quite another. At the end of the project, how many peer helpers can be retained and redeployed elsewhere? They will have built up valuable experience, which should not be wasted, if at all possible. Consider approaching clients who have received peer helping in one cycle to see if they might become peer helpers in a new cycle. How will projects be driven forward once the researchers have departed?–obviously, the role of local organizations is key here. From an evaluation perspective, you may find that longer-term results are even more powerful than short-term results (which makes it important that you look for them), and if this is the case, you will be able to make a stronger bid for more financial support for your project.

DOING MORE WITH LESS

Organizing and delivering a peer intervention might now seem somewhat more complicated than had been imagined. Particularly if you are in a developing country, you may have great difficulty delivering all 18 components described above as desirable, not least because of limitations on funding and staffing resources. However, do not be put off. The 18 components are a list of desirables, not a list of absolute requirements. There is research which shows that peer interventions can still be effective when only the sketchiest of these parameters are met. After reading this chapter, you will at least be clear about what you are not doing because you cannot, and what you might do when conditions permit to increase the effectiveness of your peer intervention.

REFERENCES

Kotera, Y., Newby, C., Charles, A., Ng, F., Watson, E., Davidson, L., et al. (2023). Typology of mental health peer support work components: Systematised review and expert consultation. *International Journal of Mental Health and Addiction.* https://doi.org/10.1007/s11469-023-01126-7

Larimer, M. E., Kilmer, J. R., Cronce, J. M., Hultgren, B. A., Gilson, M. S., & Lee, C. M. (2022). Thirty years of BASICS: Dissemination and implementation progress and challenges. *Psychology of Addictive Behaviors*, *36*(6), 664. https://doi.org/10.1037/adb0000794

Lekka, F., Efstathiou, G., & Kalantzi-Azizi, A. (2015). The effect of counselling-based training on online peer support. *British Journal of Guidance & Counselling*, *43*(1), 156–170. https://doi.org/10.1080/03069885.2014.959472

Mark, D., Lovich, R., Walker, D., Burdock, T., Ronan, A., Ameyan, W., et al. (2019). *Providing peer support for adolescents and young people living with HIV.* Child Survival Working Group. World Health Organization. www.teampata.org/pata-research/ or www.childrenandaids.org/learning-center-page

McCrary, H., Etwaroo, E., Marshall, L., Burden, E. St, Pierre, M., Berkebile, B., et al. (2022). *Peer recovery support services in correctional settings.* Bureau of Justice Assistance, US Department of Justice.

Evaluation

16

This chapter developed from an analysis of the preceding chapters. The outcome indicators could be categorized into five groups: Descriptives; Subjective Perceptions; Knowledge, Attitudes and Behavioral Intentions; Behaviors; Physiological Indicators. Importantly, peer supporters and relevant organizations should be involved in developing the tools and methods used, as well as validating them before use.

OUTCOMES–DESCRIPTIVES

These outcomes would include description of the program, for example in terms of gender focus (male, female, both), number of sessions/meetings, length of sessions/meetings, length of program, location of sessions/meetings (school, college, workplace, community center, homes, etc.), record-keeping system, monitoring arrangements, and so on. Some of these might depend on self-report by participants.

OUTCOMES–PERCEPTIONS

These outcomes would include subjective perceptions of the project from a variety of stakeholders (e.g., helper, person helped, spouse or partner of person helped, children of person helped, professional staff who have insight into the program, and so on). These can then be triangulated. Perceptions can be gathered by questionnaire, individual interview, or focus groups.

Questionnaires typically have a majority of closed questions inviting responses on some kind of scale, with a small number of open questions which will be more difficult to analyze. The scale should only have the

DOI: 10.1201/9781003438366-16

extremes adjectivally labelled, or statistical analysis will be compromised. Questions should not all lead the participant in one direction but be in randomized directions. Questionnaires are increasingly given digitally, but this may not be sensible in areas where access to devices and the internet is poor.

If the participants are in any way vulnerable, individual interviews will usually seem more sensitive, but participants may be less likely to volunteer for interview than questionnaire. Some sort of interview schedule will be needed, even if only semi-structured. In any event, interviews take longer to analyze than questionnaires, and some random sampling to identify a smaller number of potential participants will be necessary.

Focus groups gather together six to ten participants, but ideally, these should be randomly selected rather than self-selected volunteers. A timescale and a few preliminary questions should be given beforehand, with further questions in the meeting. Expect different and contrary views. Recording the session will be necessary as it will take some time to analyze. Perceptions should be assessed before and after the intervention, and preferably at follow-up also. The perceptions of a non-intervened comparison group may also be useful, although questions asked of them would be fewer than for intervened participants.

OUTCOMES–KNOWLEDGE, ATTITUDES AND BEHAVIORAL INTENTIONS

Peer education is principally about increasing knowledge, and this can be tested by pre-post knowledge tests. Peer counseling and support, by contrast, are less about knowledge and more about changes in attitudes and intention to behave differently. These are much more slippery to measure and may largely depend on self-report. Participants' attitude to themselves is also significant, and this may be described as self-confidence or self-efficacy.

Outcomes identified in the preceding chapters include:

Knowledge: improved nutrition knowledge (including among other stakeholders than the participant), improved anti-coagulant knowledge, improved knowledge in general, knowledge of HIV status.
Attitudes: reduced distress, reduced depression, reduced anxiety, reduced feelings of uncertainty and isolation, improved quality-of-life, improved psychological wellbeing, improved self-efficacy, improved satisfaction with various life domains, improved sense of community belonging, improved sense of new meaning and purpose in life, development of a new self-identity, increasing feelings of belonging and satisfaction from life, increased satisfaction with treatment experience.

Behavioral intentions: intention to increase screening implementation, change dietary intake behaviors, increase physical activity, improve ability to access resources, improve self-management, improve self-care, improve goal setting, improve problem solving, increase hope, increase control, increase ability to effect changes in their lives, reduce HIV risk behavior, take an HIV test, improved capacity to disclose HIV status to intimate partner, improved capacity to use protective practices, stronger commitment to avoid crime.

OUTCOMES–BEHAVIORS

Behaviors are things that participants actually do in response to the intervention, or an increase or decrease in pre-existing behaviors. Again, there may be some dependence on self-report, but again attempts should be made to gather data from a variety of sources (e.g., helper, person helped, spouse or partner of person helped, children of person helped, professional staff who have insight into the program, and so on). These can then be triangulated. Where the outcome is a change in behavior, pre-intervention measures of behavior are needed to compare with during-intervention and post-intervention measures. In these circumstances, additional pre-post comparison with a non-intervened group is valuable.

Behavior outcomes included age at sexual debut, condom use, unprotected sex, frequency of intercourse, initiation of sexual activity, number of sexual partners, frequency of HIV testing, unprotected anal intercourse, use of contraception, reduced equipment sharing among injection users, water-based lubricant use, reduced use of recreational drugs and alcohol before sex, reduced HIV incidence and prevalence, increased service access, changed risk behaviors, reduced stigma and discrimination, CD4 testing, antiretroviral therapy (ART) adherence, retention in HIV care, uptake of HIV testing, reduction in hepatitis C virus infection, ongoing HIV transmission, risk appraisals, viral suppression, greater confidence with health professionals, significant reduction in systolic blood pressure, decrease in amount of alcohol consumed, fewer depressive symptoms, fewer underweight infants, significantly more likely to exclusively breastfeed infants for at least six months, reduced stillbirth, breast cancer screening uptake, reduced anxiety, reduced fatigue, reduced nausea/vomiting, medication adherence, reduced pain, fewer emergency room visits, reduction in hospital readmission rate, improved daily living activities, improved limb function, unplanned readmissions, improved self-efficacy, reduced depressive symptoms up to 180 days post-discharge, satisfaction with life at 180 days, reduction in use of emergency rooms, reducing substance use, hospitalization days, total medical costs, abstaining from alcohol, reducing alcohol use, quantity and frequency of drinking, estimated peak blood alcohol concentration, reducing alcohol-related consequences, reduction in students drunk for the first time, binge-drinking, reduced relapse rates, improved relationships with treatment providers, reduced substance use, reduced human immunodeficiency virus/hepatitis C virus risk behaviors, reduced craving, less frequent injection, decline in injection risk, better access to methadone and HIV clinics. reduction in smoking, biochemically verified seven-day abstinence at three months, reduced consumption of drugs, more quit attempts, abstinence at follow-up –three to nine months later, improved behavior, improved diet, improved physical activity, improved body measures, improved body weight, improved body mass index (BMI), improved waist circumference, significant increase in physical activity, improved discontinuing breast feeding, improved dietary pattern, improved fruit and vegetable intake, reduced fat intake, reduced complementary feeding, increased minimum meal frequency, increased dietary diversity, exclusive breastfeeding, reduced risk of opioid overdose, reduced self-injury, reduced anti-coagulant complication rates, improved anti-coagulant therapy compliance, improved use of antithrombotic medications at six months, reduced relapse rates, increased treatment retention, reduced overdosing, improved enrolment in methadone clinics, improved enrolment in HIV clinics, improvement in pedometer measures, improvement in accelerometry, improvement in step count, reduction of purchase of biscuits and ice cream, weekly duration of physical activity, weekly frequency of physical activity, breastfeeding initiation, breastfeeding duration, breastfeeding exclusivity, reduced infant diarrhea, increased lactational amenorrhea, exclusive breastfeeding duration, breastfeeding within the first hour of life, pre-lacteal feeding, reduced self-harm, reduced suicide attempts, reduced sexual assault, reduced violence, reduced needle sharing, reduced injecting, reduced re-offending up to 16 months later, increased uptake of sexually transmitted infection (STI) and bloodborne viruses (BBV) testing, reduced bullying, drug abstinence, reduced smartphone addiction, reduced head lice infestation, reduced social isolation, improved access to public services.

OUTCOMES–PHYSIOLOGICAL INDICES

Physiological indices are arguably the most "objective" way of measuring outcomes, but there is still the problem of participants presenting themselves for regular testing, which has a cost in terms of participant time.

"Testing fatigue" may set in after a while and testing frequencies decline. Thus, required testing needs to be set at reasonable limits from the outset. If testing can be done during home visits or very locally to the participant, so much the better.

Physiological outcomes include reduced chlamydia infection, reduced STI, reduced prevalence of bacterial STIs (chlamydia, gonorrhea, trichomonas, and syphilis), improved glycemic control (HbA1c), improved blood pressure, improved diastolic blood pressure, improved cholesterol levels, improved BMI, significant reduction in average blood glucose (sugar) levels, improved fasting blood sugar, improved HbA1c cholesterol, improved high density cholesterol, reduced weight, reduced smoking, quit smoking, improved diet, increased physical activity, improved low-density lipoprotein, improved other lipids, improved foot care, reduced waist circumference, improved lung function, peak blood alcohol content, HIV antibody testing, reduced rates of hepatitis B, HCV antibody testing, improved HCV serology tests, improved mobile elastography reduced exhaled carbon monoxide, biochemically verified seven-day smoking abstinence, improved salivary cotinine test, improved tuberculosis, improvement in liver disease.

COMBINATIONS OF OUTCOME MEASURES

It follows that a combination of outcome measures would be most likely to give an accurate picture. Ideally, researchers should take one outcome measure from each of the five categories above (or more, if possible, but do not be too ambitious and over-commit). There may well be differences between outcomes from different categories (e.g., very positive perceptions but no change in physiological indices). All will need describing fully in the final report.

REMAINING ISSUES

Remaining questions relate to comparisons between peer-led and professional-led services, cost-effectiveness and long-term follow-up.

In several chapters, the research evidence shows that peer-led interventions performed as well as or better than professional-led interventions.

Peers were better able to reduce inpatient use and improve a range of recovery outcomes. Peer services were generally equally effective to services provided by non-peer paraprofessionals on traditional clinical outcomes. Peer-delivered interventions were just as effective as professionally delivered interventions for increasing physical activity. However, in fact, this comparison is less than helpful, as peer-led interventions need support from professional services if they are to function effectively. This would of course require some change in how the professional services characterize their job function.

Turning to cost-effectiveness, in at least one area, peer-led education was more cost-effective than professionally led education for the prevention of HIV infection. However, again this finding is somewhat illusory. Many more studies need to give a detailed account of cost-effectiveness, with realistic accounting for the time of peer helpers and the time of supporting health professionals.

More long-term follow-up is required if the research literature is to stand as robust and peer intervention is to be seen as sustainable. While peer interventions may shift and metamorphose as their supporting organizations come and go, at least more evidence is required of longer-term sustainability of gains from intervention, although the expectations here should be realistic.

Discussion and Conclusion 17

LIMITATIONS AND STRENGTHS

Readers might have been surprised that no attempt was made to assess the quality of the reviews mentioned in these chapters. There were a number of reasons for that. Firstly, the quality of studies was in general higher from developed countries than developing countries (although with some notable exceptions), so any assessment would have been somewhat unfair in that respect. Secondly, the quality of studies from both developed and developing countries tended to increase as time went by, so later studies were more likely to be of good quality. Thirdly, the definition of "good quality" is itself a contentious term. For some, "good quality" means randomized controlled trials (RCTs). Others note that RCTs often focus on a very small number of studies, ignoring most of the literature in the area. Yet, others would argue that quantitative positivistic methods can never convey the richness of what is being researched. On the other hand, purely qualitative researchers have difficulty making claims about outcomes, as they only have subjective perceptions to rely on.

One might naively assume that as reviews (especially systematic reviews and meta-analyses) follow a standard pattern, they are comparable. However, inspection of any of the preceding chapters shows very quickly that even these are very variable—in terms of the keywords chosen for the search, the time range of the search, the number and type of databases searched and the inclusion criteria for studies. Given this, it is perhaps surprising that there is as much agreement between them as is actually seen.

The single studies chosen for inclusion were selected on the basis of being in developed or developing countries (examples in both being required). They tended to be relatively recent, and a balance was attempted between different kinds of study. However, the decision was an intuitive one by the author. These single studies were merely examples of what was available, rather than anything more representative. The exemplar single study reported in detail regarding implementation was again chosen intuitively by the author. These again tended to be relatively recent, alternating from developed to developing country from one chapter to the next. Remarkably, few studies in each chapter gave enough detail about implementation to be considered for inclusion.

Regarding the reviews and studies themselves, in relatively few cases was longer-term follow-up part of the project. Thus, we do generally not know if there were any enduring effects. Of course, it might not be reasonable to expect enduring effects, especially if the intervention is stopped, since many other life events will intervene and cloud the picture. Nonetheless, some degree of sustainability of outcomes, both with continuing intervention and without it, would be welcome. Those projects which have continuity arrangements, with clients in receipt of service being recruited to be new peer helpers, clearly have advantages here, not least since there is evidence of benefit to peer helpers as well as the helped (although we have not reviewed this evidence here).

Turning to discuss strengths, the main strength is the sheer volume of reviews and single studies discovered. Although only a few single studies were reported, the list of relevant single studies for each chapter forms a rich online resource which readers may wish to search not just by chapter title but also by keywords of their particular interest. It is evident that some chapters report far more research than others, and of course, there are other areas where there is so little research that there is no chapter under that heading. It is interesting to see what topics appear to be fashionable (and consequently, what not) and what the balance between developed and developing countries is.

The other strength is the focus here not just on outcomes, but also on implementation–i.e., how that outcome was achieved and in what context. Knowledge of "what works" is all very well, but it is only the first step towards delivering services that make a difference. For this latter, detailed awareness of how to implement in any specific context is needed, and project leaders need to be sharply aware of the importance of constant re-adjustment to meet developing challenges during the course of the project.

SUMMARY OF RESULTS

Regarding Sexual Health, there were 19 reviews of evidence. Six of these were concerned with youth and adolescence, five with school- and college-based programs, four with developing countries (general, Iran, India and

South-east Asia), three with LGBT populations and one with digital sexual health. Knowledge and attitude changes were very common, and (particularly more recently) higher quality studies had found objective evidence of effects. There were 87 single studies, 39 in developed countries and 48 (55%) in developing countries, reflecting the degree of concern in developing countries. Just a few showed no intervention effects.

There were 38 reviews of peer interventions with HIV/AIDS. Fourteen of these (37%) came from or referred to developing countries. Almost all reviews found that most studies showed peer intervention to be effective, especially later reviews. There were 146 single studies; 96 of these (66%) came from or referred to developing countries or disadvantaged groups.

There were 29 reviews of research on peer interventions for Cancer. Ten dealt with specific kinds of cancer, 14 with all types. Reviews generally found interventions effective at moderate levels, although a few studies were neural or negative. There was also evidence of post-traumatic psychological growth from cancer. Online peer support by itself showed mixed effectiveness. There were 100 single studies; 33 of these (33%) explored preventive approaches, while 67 focused on corrective measures. While for preventive studies the proportion of studies from developing countries was similar to that for other medical conditions, for corrective studies, this proportion was much lower.

Peer intervention for people with diabetes has been very extensively researched. Twenty-seven reviews of research were identified. Some reviews reported a high average impact on glycemic control (HbA1c), other reviews a smaller impact, and other reviews improvement only in some studies. Some studies also showed improvements in blood pressure, cholesterol and body mass index (BMI)/weight. Overall, 126 single studies were identified. Effects were more likely with higher frequency of contact and intervention for three to six months was most effective. Three reviews investigated developing countries: two were positive with improvements in HbA1c, blood pressure and BMI. Four technology-based interventions were identified: phone-based text messages, video, web portal and social media. Mixed findings were observed in reduced HbA1c levels.

Chapter 6 focused on chronic health conditions; heart, neurological and other conditions; spinal cord injury, stroke and asthma. There were 34 reviews of evidence, 11 in chronic health conditions, eight spinal cord injury, four in heart conditions, four in neurological conditions, two in stroke and two in asthma. Reviews in chronic health conditions were positive; most studies reported improvement compared to controls in most if not all outcomes, although studies of digital technology and in low- and middle-income countries were less certain. Spinal cord injury interventions were a little less successful, but still made a significant difference. Heart condition reviews were generally very positive. Neurological reviews were again not so strong, but still showed improvements in a majority of studies and a majority of outcomes. Reviews for stroke were again very positive. For asthma, the reviews were least positive, generally showing only small non-significant improvement for the intervention group. There were six single studies on chronic health conditions, 18 on spinal cord injury, 32 on heart conditions, four on stroke and ten on asthma.

Concerning mental health, there were 40 reviews of evidence, the great majority on mental health in general, but some with an emphasis on adolescence/youth and schools/universities. Five focused on depression including suicide prevention and one on schizophrenia. Early studies had mixed results but later studies more consistently positive results, although still with some negative findings. Studies of young people and adults both had similar results. Peer intervention seemed particularly effective with depression but less effective with schizophrenia. There were 81 individual studies; 59 concerned general mental health and nine concerned depression. Autism, bullying, eating disorders, schizophrenia and suicide prevention all had two papers. Only five papers (out of 81, 6%) were from developing countries, with a further four targeting minority populations in developed countries.

There were six reviews of peer intervention in alcohol abuse, but only half focused wholly on this topic and two of these were only with university/college students. School-based peer education showed mixed results, while some programs with university/college students were more effective. There were 14 single studies from developed countries and three from developing countries.

There were 11 reviews of research on drug use and abuse. Positive effects included reduced relapse rates, increased treatment retention, improved relationships with treatment providers and social supports, increased satisfaction with the overall treatment experience, reduced substance use, reduced human immunodeficiency virus/hepatitis C virus risk behaviors, reduced craving and increased self-efficacy. There was occasional mention of null findings. There were 26 single studies, of which 19 were in developed countries and seven in developing countries. These found a decline in injection risk, more frequent condom use, higher retention and better access to methadone and HIV clinics.

Smoking had eight reviews of research. Early reviews found more studies showing improvement in smoking than otherwise. Some reviews measured ancillary variables such as self-efficacy rather than actual smoking reduction. The most recent review showed effectiveness across 15 studies and included follow-up at up to nine months. Effect sizes were greatest among interventions with formerly smoking peers as helpers. Turning to the 48 single studies of smoking, there were 73% in a developed country and 27% in a developing country.

Interventions to increase physical activity have become more widespread, to prevent or reduce obesity. There were seven reviews on obesity and ten on physical activity. Six reviews on obesity had mainly positive results, but one on obesity in mental health was more negative. Reviews of physical activity interventions found about two-thirds of them had positive outcomes, and overall effect sizes were moderate, but higher in studies with follow-up. There were 39 single studies on obesity and 46 on physical activity. In obesity, 14 out of 39 studies (36%) were from developing countries or focused on disadvantaged communities. In physical activity, six out of 46 studies (13%) were from developing countries or focused on disadvantaged communities.

Several reviews of breastfeeding and nutrition focused on low- and middle-income countries. There were 24 reviews of evidence on breastfeeding. Peer intervention seemed effective, particularly in the antenatal period and in low- and middle-income countries. Peer intervention combined with professional support seemed most effective. There were nine reviews of nutrition. Peer intervention was generally effective, although studies in schools were more likely to use only subjective evidence. Both home visits and group-based methods were effective. Social media interventions in schools could be effective.

Peer interventions actually within prisons were considered, rather than peer interventions for released prisoners as well. Much of the work here was about HIV/AIDS prevention and treatment (also see Chapter 3), drug abuse (also see Chapter 9) and suicide prevention (also see Chapter 7). There were 14 reviews of evidence, mostly general reviews of peer intervention in all conditions, plus two reviews of peer intervention in HIV/AIDS, one on self-injury and one on sexual offenders. Effects on attitudes, knowledge and behavioral intentions regarding HIV risk behavior were commonly found. Being a peer deliverer was associated with positive effects on the deliverer. There were 36 single studies. Eleven concerned general effects of peer intervention. Nine of them concerned HV/AIDS. Six focused on hepatitis C. Turning to mental health, there were two studies, two on self-harm and one on suicide prevention. Beyond this, there were two studies on drug abuse. Finally, there were two studies on tuberculosis (both from Ethiopia).

Other areas of interest were not searched for but cropped up in other searches. There were five reviews. Three of these were reviews of peer intervention in social isolation, but the results were not that encouraging. Four out of five studies found community interventions plus health facilities had an effect.

CONCLUSION

There was strong evidence of the effectiveness of peer intervention in Sexual Health, HIV/AIDS, Cancer (although online support was weaker), Diabetes (principally on biological indicators, although online support was again weaker), Chronic Health Conditions (digital and low- and middle-income studies again weaker), Heart Conditions, Stroke, Drug Use, Smoking, Obesity, Breastfeeding and Nutrition. There was moderate evidence of the effectiveness of peer intervention in Spinal Cord Injury, Neurological Conditions, Mental Health, Alcohol Abuse, Physical Activity (and social media interventions could be effective) and Peer Interventions within Prisons (also see Chapters 3, 7 and 9). There was weak to no evidence of the effectiveness of peer intervention in: Asthma. There were more single studies in developing countries than in developed countries in the areas of: Sexual Health, HIV/AIDS, Breastfeeding and Nutrition.

Had all studies followed the practice recommendations made in Chapters 15 and 16 of this book, it may be that the strength of evidence would have improved for the moderate and weak areas, as well as generating better evidence on new areas not yet mentioned here. However, following all those recommendations would have increased cost (even assuming it were possible), which raises the issue of cost-effectiveness. Peer intervention may be cheaper than professional intervention, but it is not free, not least since professional time is taken up with organizing, operating and monitoring the intervention. Additionally, peer intervention may occur more frequently than professional intervention, albeit at lower unit cost. A few studies did address the issue of cost-effectiveness, but in such varied contexts that they were difficult to summarize. There is no doubt that cost-effectiveness and longer-term follow-up are the two questions urgently needing more research.

Index

Note: Page numbers in **bold** refer to tables.